How to Eat Cock
The Sofa King Easy Way!

The essential cookbook for eating cock, clams, wieners, beaver and more!

by
Kristy Kream

Copyrigt ©2020, Sofa King Rad, LLC
All Rights Reserved.

THIS IS A PARODY!

DISCLAIMER!!!

Let it be known that you (the buyer(s)) are hereby notified that the How to Eat Cock, The Sofa King East Way is an all-out parody. It's full of Bad spelling, grammar, not very funny tasteless jokes, and truly tasteful recipes! They're unedited, unruly, raw and may contain material not suitable for areas outside your own kitchen. You have been officially notified!

Copyright ©2020 by Sofa King Rad.

All rights reserved. This book or any portion thereof may not be reproduced or used in any manner whatsoever without the express written permission of the publisher except for the use of brief quotations in a book review.

Fourth Edition, First Printing, 2020 in the United States of America

Sofa King Rad Publishing
1127 Quivira Dr.
Colorado Springs, CO 80910
ISBN 978-1-7361214-5-0
www.SofaKingRad.com

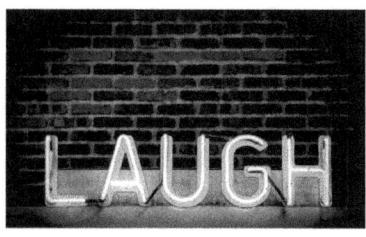

"This book is a parody. If you don't think eating cock is funny... go back to eating pussy!"
  -G Wilson, Los Angeles

This is a parody cookbook. These are just jokes folks! Don't be afraid to laugh even if you have never eaten a rooster before in your life!

Our goal is to help you get past your Alektorophobia right now and to get you to start enjoying eating cock *The Sofa King Easy Way.*

We here at Sofa King Easy, know that people take their cock-eating very seriously. In fact, we know a few highly experienced cock eaters that could write novels on the subject. Our goal is to make your cock eating more fun, fulfilling, and tasty for everyone.

This book is packed full of pleasantly pungent puns, grammar only a grandma could love, totally tasteless jokes, and some handy (pardon the pun) tasteful recipes.

A kaleidoscope of fun for all except for older folks, kids, dogs, some cats, religious fanatics or anyone who doesn't enjoy eating hot cock. You know who you are!

DISCOUNTS & CONTESTS ON MORE SOFA KING EASY BOOKS FOR FRIENDS AND LOTS OF OTHER SOFA KING FREE STUFF!!!

JOIN OUR FACEBOOK SOFA KING EASY FAN PAGE

Thank you for buying our Sofa King Easy Book and not stealing it from someone. As a reward, we want to give you a discount coupon for your next *"How to Eat Cock the Sofa King Easy Way"* cookbook. Perhaps you could buy one to replace the one you just stole???

There are contests for the best photo, video and more ways to get famous!

$ $ $ $ $ $ $ $ $

GO NOW AND GET YOUR COUPON!!!
Before whoever you stole this from finds out their copy is missing!

$ $ $ $ $ $ $ $ $

GO TO:
Facebook: Sofa King Rad
Web: sofakingrad.com

If you have any problems or have something to contribute and cant spel email me at:
support@sofakingrad.com

HOW TO EAT COCK
THE SOFA KING EASY WAY!

Disclaimer!!! 2
Discounts & Contests on more Sofa King Easy books for Friends and Lots of Other Sofa King Free Stuff!!! 4
    Join Our Facebook Sofa King Easy Fan Page 4
Forward 13
Cock, Rooster & 15
Other Foul Things 15
    Preparing Your Cock 16
        Wash your Cock 16
        Get Your Meat Read 16
        #1 Beat Your Meat 16
        #2 Pound Your Meat 17
        #3 Age Your Meat 17
    Your Cock Tips 17
    Beer Butt Cock 19
        Bottoms Up Bar & Grill 19
        Gaylordsville, Connecticut 19
    Drunk Cock 23
        Kum Den 23
        Uncertain, TX 23
    Exploding Cock 26
        Wiener's Circle 26
        Pee Pee, Ohio 26
    Lardon Coq Au Vin 27
        Phat Phuc Noodle Bar 27
        Imalone, Wisconsin 27
    Slow Jerky Jamaica Cock 29
        Jamaica-MiKrazY Restaurant 29
        Uman Hole St. Andrew 29
    Fast Jerky Asian Cock 31
        Fu King Chinese Restaurant 31
        Pee-King China 31
    Bar-B-Que'd BBC 33
        Eat Me 33
        Snakebite Ridge, Texas 33

Cockpot-A- Doodle Doo 35
    Peking Inn 35
    Kickapoo, Kansas 35
Crock Pot Cocky Cream Pie 37
    Life of Pie 37
    Pie Town, New Mexico 37
Cock 'N Bull Stew 39
    Nuts and Screws Burger Pit 39
    Hell, Michigan 39
Elephant Cock Stew 41
    The African Café 41
Crock Pot "Cock 'n Bull" Stew 43
    Happy Crack 43
    Double Cross, NV. 43
Captain Jack Alfredo's Flat Cock 45
    Happy Daze 45
    Holetown, Barbados 45
Smoking Cock 48
    Lord of the Fries 48
    Los Baños, CA. 48
Cock Sammich 50
    Bite Me Sandwiches 50
    Greenwich Village, NY 50

Cow **52**
Slow Cow Tongue 53
    Brad's Pit 53
    Wichita, KS. 53
Cow Love Sticks 55
    Gay Johnson's 55
    Grand Junction, CO. 55
Beef Cheek Tacos 57
    Tacos de Cabeza on The Plaza 57
    Bucerias, Mexico 57
Cow Stroganoff 60
    Phat Dong 60
    Screamer, Alabama 60
Bitchin' Brazed Cow Tails 62
    Happy Tails to You 62
    Until we Meat Again Cafe   Smackover, Utah 62
Udder Butter Cream 64
    Cheesy Does It 64
    Slickpoo, ID. 64

Chicken **66**
Dirty Rice – Dirty Chicken 67

- Itchy Butt Chicken and Joy 67
  - Tightwad, MO. 67
- Aunt Fred's Breaded Chicken Arms 69
  - Anal Indian Takeaway 69
  - Tulsa, Ok. 69
- Lime Chicken & Sticky Honey Sauce 71
  - Wok This Way! 71
  - Boston, MA 71
- Sticky Honey Breasts 73
  - El Arroyo 73
  - Spread eagle, WI 73
- Chicken Breasts & Creamy BBC 75
  - Lick a Chick Restaurant 75
  - Eel Pie Island, River Thames 75
- Big Breasts –N- Taquitos 77
  - Whadda Lookin' At?! Food Truck 77
  - New York, NY (down by da docks) 77

Clams & Oysters 80
- Hot Noodle Deep in White Clam Sauce 81
  - The Munch Box 81
  - Virgin, Utah 81
- RMO (Rocky Mountain Oysters) 84
  - Stoner's Paradise 84
  - Loveland, Colorado 84
- Drunken Clams & Sausage 86
  - My Fucking Restaurant 86
  - Cincinnati, Ohio 86
- Beer Steamed Clams 88
  - Eat Me 88
  - Cincinnati, Ohio 88
- Long Dong Squirt & Tequila 90
  - Long Dong Silvers 90
  - Ballsalla 90
  - Isle Of Man 90

Wieners, Tube Steaks & Other Low Hanging Meats 93
- Sheboygan Slammers 94
  - the Sheboygan Slammer Queen 94
  - Sheboygan, WI 94
- Mac's & Jack's BIG Creamy Slammers 96
  - Like No Udder 96
  - Milwaukee, Wisconsin 96
- How's Your AssBeen? 98
- (Smokin' Hot Round Bottoms) 98
  - Slope Side Meets 98
  - Aspen, Colorado 98

Korean BBQ Meat Doll 100
    Just Falafs 100
    Keister, West Virginia 100
Perfect Prime Rib 101
    Spex In The City 101
    Florida Keys. FL 101
Roger Rabbit Ragu 104
    Lettuce Eat 104
    Bangalore, India 104
Mushroom Head Teriyaki Skewers 106
    Gochew Grill 106
    Truth Or Consequences, New Mexico 106
Loin Knockers With Small Onions 108
    Hung Far Low 108
    Mock City, Washington 108
Mr. Big's Skin Flutes 110
    Late Night Dine Right 110
    San Francisco, CA. 110
BIG Jim and the Twins 112
    Chops & Hops 112
    Two Wallnuts, Florida 112
Little Willies 114
    Two Men and a Griddle 114
    Embarrass, MN. 114
Wrap That Weiner 116
    Thai Me Up Restaurant & Brewery Protection, KS. 116
Black & Blue Little Berries Yogurt Sauce 118
    Black & Blue Berries Café 118
    Shushup, Wi. 118
Slow-Cooker Beer Brats 120
    Wish you were Beer 120
    Hempstead, NY 120
Beer Cheese Beer Beefy Brats and Beer 122
    Bacon Bros. Diner 122
    Redwing MN. 122
Wrapped Mini-wieners 124
    The Munchy Queen 124
    Plano, Texas 124
Bite size Whiskey wieners 126
    Hangover Cure 126
    Accident, Maryland 126
Beaver **128**
    Shaved Asian Beavers 129
        Fuckoffee 129
        Cut And Shoot, Texas 129

S&M's Tender Beaver 131
    Thai Me Up 131
    Frustrated, Oklahoma 131
One Drunk Beaver 133
    Custards Last Stand 133
    Somefield SD. 133
Can Do Beaver 135
    Decadent Desire 135
    Las Vegas, Nevada 135
Rosie's Giant Pink Corn Taco & White Cream Sauce 136
    The Pink Taco Van 136
    South Side Los Angeles, CA. 136
Pho King Beaver Bangers 138
    Pho King Good Noodles 138
    Truth or Consequences, NM. 138

Rubs, Sauces, Stews & Soups 140
  Your Rubing Tips 141
  Rub One Out On Your Street Tacos 142
    Burrito Belly 142
    Hippo, Kentucky 142
  "I'm On a Dry Rub to Hell!" (sing it!) 143
    Uncle Tony's House 143
    Cleveland, Ohio 143
  Turbo's Coffee Bean Rub 145
    Barnyard Breakfast Diner & Automat 145
    Chicken, Alaska 145
  Ewe Rub, I Rub, We Rub 147
    Mother Cluckers 147
    Hazard, Nebraska 147
  Dirty Dick's! (rub sauce) 149
    Dirty Dick's Crab House 149
    St. Petersburg, FL. 149
  Peter's Thick White Sauce 151
    Filled of dreams 151
    Intercourse, PA. 151
  Who's Your Daddy?! Slap Sauce 153
    Nacho Daddy's Grill 153
    Knockemstiff, Ohio 153
  Cuz' I'm Your Mother and I said so!! 155
    Nacho Daddy 155
    Knockemstiff, Ohio 155
  Marley's Smokin' Oh Juice 157
    Jamaica Mi Krazy Kafe 157
    Mexican Water, AZ. 157
  Soup for the Dead 159

Nin Com Soup 159
   Caca Del Toro, Mexico 159
Leekie Cock Soup 161
   Thai Tanic Restaurant 161
   Toledo, Ohio 161
Happy Onions in Herbs Ball Sack 163
   Town Cry Here Onion Bar 163
   Sheep Boot, Ma. 163

Sofa King Faking It 165
Worlds Best Yakitori Sauce 166
& Chicken Skewers 166
   Yakitori 166
   Colorado Springs, Colorado 166
   Chicken skewers: 167
KFC's Original Fried Chicken 168
Star Bucks egg bites 171
White Castle Sliders 173
Steve's Sweet and Salty Hot Nuts 175
Orange Julius 177

Side Kicks! 178
Emo Philip's Coleslaw Recipe 179
   By Emo Philips 179
Dirty Tater Bites 181
   I Dream of Weenie 181
   Baked, Alaska 181
Great Head Job 182
   (Sautéed mushrooms) 182
   The Golden Spoon Café 182
   Darnkids, Florida 182
Momma-T's Tater Tot Casserole 184
   Momma-T's 184
   Bumpass, Va. 184

Appetizers (first bites) 187
Pass Around My Sweet, Salty & Spicy Nuts 188
   Wild Thyme Café Bar 188
   Smithville, Tn 188
Chef's Chocolate Salty Balls 190
   Chewy Balls 190
   South Park, CO 190
St. Christmas Crack Nuts 192
   Under Santa's North Pole 192
Swollen Members' Chocolate Walnut Shrimp 194
   Turnip the Beet Café 194
   Port Angeles, WA. 194
Canned Peas 196

King Soopers 196
No Name, Colorado 196
Stuff That Camel 197
Syrian Dipity 197
Dustmaskus, Syria 197
.... 198

Totally Gross Things Your Grandparents Put in Their Mouths 199
70s Diet Jellied Tomato Refresher 200
Upright Organ Party 201
Yawning in Technicolor 203
Veggie Fruit Salad 203
Spinal Tap Vertebrae Hot Dogs 206

Deserts 208
Banana Mayonnaise Candle 209
Tequila Cookies 210
Tequila Mockingbird 210
Ocean City, MD 210
Mile High Asphalt Pie 212
Denver Mint 212
Denver, Co. 212
\ 214

DRINKS 215
Buttery Nipple 216
Zip It Down Creamy Milky Surprise   Energy Drink 216
Purple-Headed Yogurt Flingers 217
Sex on the Beach 218
Blowjob 218
Liquid Viagra 219
Slippery Nipple 219
Screaming Orgasm 219
Super Slow Comfortable Screw 220
Sex Machine 220
Sit on My Face 221
Deep Throat 221
Creamy Pussy 222
Harvey Wall banger 222
Pop My Cherry 223
Bend Over Shirley 223
Three-Legged Monkey 223
Dr. Pecker 224
Penile Colarous 224
Tight Snatch 225
Bearded Clam 225
Strawberry Stripper 226

Orange Bush 226
Fuzzy Navel..226
Dirty Mother..227
Golden Shower 227
....228
Super Red Balls 228
Royal Fook...228
Suck, Bang and Blow...229
How to Eat Pussy...230
How to Eat Pussy 230
The Sofa King Easy Way!..230

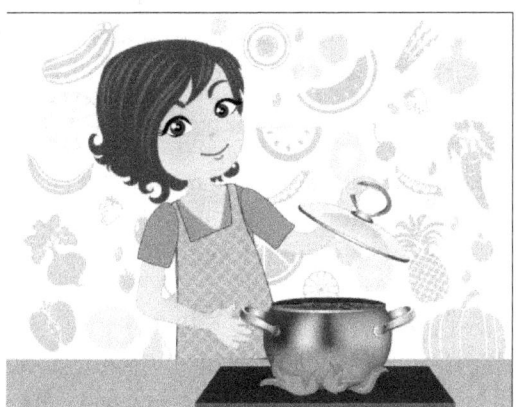

FORWARD

I remember when I got my first cock, I thought it was pretty cool. It really wasn't as ugly and scary to touch as much as I had feared.

He looked all so majestic and magnificent. I also thought it was really hilarious watching him as he was strutting his stuff all around, with his big head bobbing up and down. I knew I wanted it.

With just a little help from the farmer, I was able to catch him and hold my very first cock. As I held him up to my cheek, I knew I was in love.

When I got him back home, I really did not want to pluck him because he was so loud and obnoxious. I was genuinely terrified he would wake all the neighbors and they would see him. So, I reached into my purse, grabbed my trusty Taser, held it up to his head, and BAM! I shocked the shit out of him. My poor cock went limp immediately, dropped and plopped right onto my newly cleaned floor. I have never seen a cock go so soft so fast or a floor get so dirty so quickly.

I am often asked by my girlfriends what does a cock taste like. I have to admit that even after all the trouble of getting all dressed up to go out to find a suitable cock, talking it up all night and then finally getting it home and preparing it, that I am still afraid to taste any of them for the first time.

I am always worried it will be gamey tasting if it was not cleaned right or it would be too salty. They all taste different depending on what they eat. I prefer free-range cocks that have been fed something sweet like pineapples.

The first time I tried eating cock. I knew immediately it would be one of my favorite things to eat for the rest of my life. I can now proudly say I have eaten hundreds of cocks from all over the world.

In this book, you will learn *How to Eat Cock the Sofa King Easy Way*. Follow along with me as I revisit some of my fondest memories of eating cocks, their many creamy sauces, and the other fowl things I have put in my mouth across these United States and the world.

As I always say; any cock will do! But remember though, sooner or later you will have to talk to the cock you decide to bring home.

-Kristy Kream

"*Your body is not a temple, it's an amusement park. Enjoy the ride.*"
   —***Anthony Bourdain.***

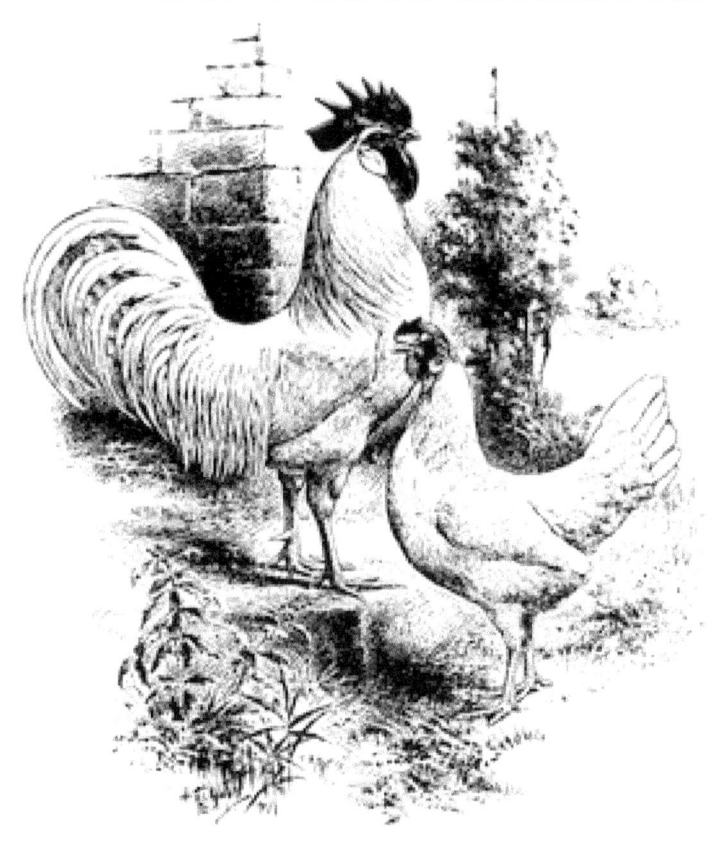

Cock, Rooster & Other Foul Things

Look, I like cock as much as anyone else. There is something about exotic meats that gets me so excited. I can really get my mouth all wet and worked up about it. Heck, I have even given beaver a try.

"While farmers generally allow one rooster for ten hens, ten men are scarcely sufficient to service one woman."
   -Giovanni Boccaccio

Preparing Your Cock

Wash your Cock
For many people, washing your cock is an essential step that must take place before they get to the fun of actually eating your cock. In a 2015 study based on a nationally representative sample of 1,504 people, 69 percent of respondents reported rinsing or washing their cocks. 31% don't care or were drunk enough not to notice.

Get Your Meat Ready
Some people think the harder a cock is at the beginning the better and to just dive right in.

Other's prefer just to start right off with a soft cock.

Globally throughout millennia, people have found some very innovative ways to solve the age old problem of hard cocks and making them soft.

There are many ways to soften up your cock. Here are just a few:

#1 Beat Your Meat
Anybody that has owned a cock for more than 15 years knows they can really take a beating.

The oldest, most natural, and most obvious way to get your cock soft is to beat it into submission by hand. The more enjoyable way is to beat it into submission with someone else's hand.

Fast Fact: It is a sad fact that 89% of cock beatings worldwide are by hand, self-inflicted, and happen with no witnesses.

#2 Pound Your Meat

Another way to soften up your cock is to pound the crap out of it. You can get your wife to wrap it in saran wrap and beat it with a rolling pin.

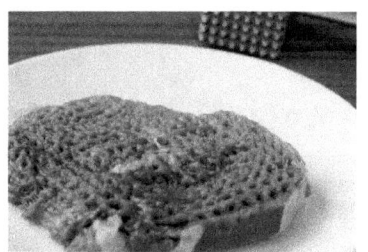

You can use a can of food, a meat hammer, a baseball bat or a heavy skillet. Anything that's hard will do.

#3 Age Your Meat

The third way to soften up a cock is by aging it. This is the least desirable of the three methods because it takes a very long time to do, and it is irreversible.

Fast Fact: Mariage is the leading cause of soft cocks.

Your Cock Tips

After I pound my cock, I put the head, back, neck, and legs into the pot and cover it with the water I used to rinse my cock with.

I simmer my cock gently for a day. Then I strain and refrigerate my cock bones and all. When pull out my cock and pick at the meat on my bone I can get a surprising amount of it off of the back, wings, and the neck.

After you get rid of your bone put your meat back in the fridge to make it get soft. Pull it out again if you are ready to make something like a cock cream pie with a super crusty bottom.

You can feed any remaining scraps to your dog or cat. They'll love you forever! Be careful when feeding a bone to a dog, though, they are known to get them stuck in their throat.

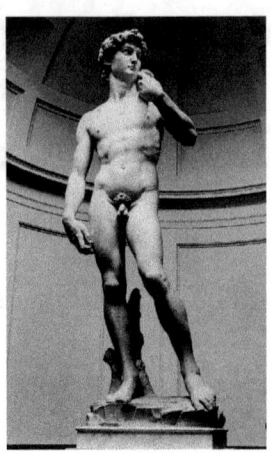

COCK

Facts are facts, and I have found out through my many years eating cock is that the young cocks are always better cocks. Old cocks are tougher cocks. Any true cock coinsurer and all of my friends will tell you just that.

To make a tough cock soft, it takes a lot of moisturizing. So much so that rubbing the cream into your cock that you can sprain a wrist! Be sure to switch your "moisturizing" hand often.

"I've heard of all sorts of ways to beat your meat; by hand mostly but I've heard of using a rolling pin, unopened cans of food and some even use hammers!

Some people beat their meat so loudly that the neighbors complain, but it's not them that are having to deal with a rock hard cock is it?"
   *-**Becky Simmons**, Hotlipp Arizona*

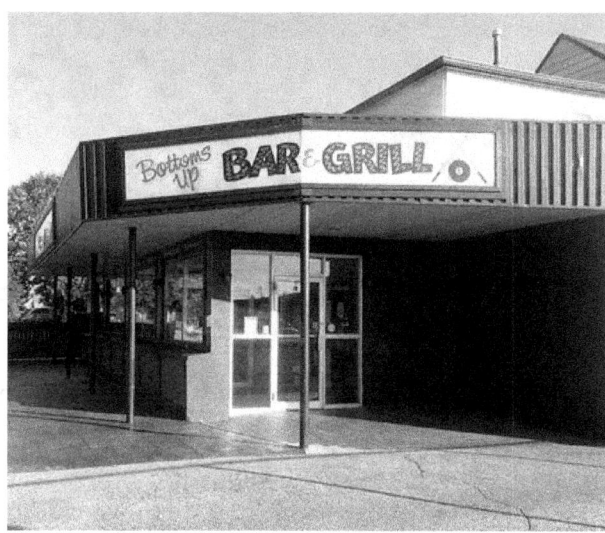
tripadvisor.com

Beer Butt Cock
Bottoms Up Bar & Grill
Gaylordsville, Connecticut

"I remember the first time I cruised Bottoms. I just had to get one of those wonderful Beer Butt Cocks into my mouth and down my throat. One of the greatest pleasures in life is eating a cock full of a great tasting beer.

I have made this recipe many times over the years, and this is my favorite way to eat cock. My husband and I have tried garlic and herb spices, lemon pepper, BBQ seasoning etc. You name it we've tried it in our cock rub.

A few words of advice: get a beer butt cock holder. It makes it easier to get the beer into your cock and rub on it.

The style of beer and the amount in the cock is really all up to the person that is going to eat it. Some prefer a good dry cock and should therefore use a smaller 12-ounce beer. If you like your meat really, really moist use, a 16-ounce beer.

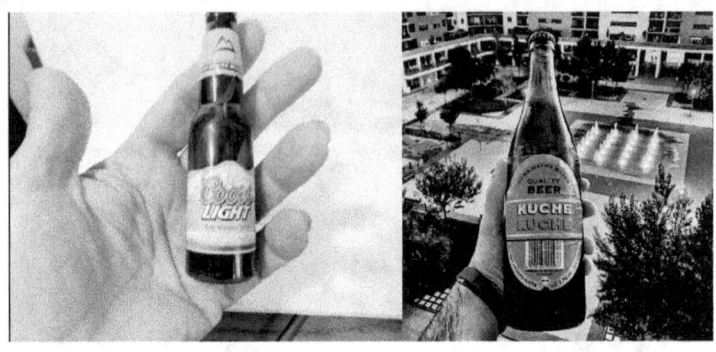

Personally, I don't think it matters much what beer you use. But some big cock coinsures swear they can tell the difference between a cock full of a wimpy golden German beer like Coors Light and a heavy, large, dark, thick South African Kuche Kuche lager from Malawi. But you know me. Domestic or imported? Who cares! As long as I have Beer Butt Cock in my mouth, I'm mega happy!

You do have to be wary of using a lot of salty seasonings when you rub your cock. Some think a cock is salty enough by itself. I'd suggest something with a little bit of spice such as a Cajun or Creole rub. Mix it with a little bit of salad oil to get the rub to stick to your cock.

Taking the temp of your cock is about what you would think. You must try to get the thermometer tip into the thicker part of your cock to measure its temp. Make sure you aren't going too far in and hitting the bottom, it can often be hotter than your cock.

The slower you cook your cock, the moister and tender it will be, just like when cooking most chicken or turkey. Make sure you do it over indirect heat. A 4lb cock usually takes about 55 minutes at ~375 degrees on the grill to release all of its juicy, creamy goodness.

Ingredients:
1 huge 4lb cock
1 can lager (I just used one pilsner but got a case of 'em.)
3 cloves of garlic
5-8 slices of bacon

Rub Ingredients:
1 tbsp onion powder
1 tbsp fresh ground black pepper
2 tsp of Mexican oregano
1 tsp of smoked paprika (I tried this in high school.)
1 tsp of ground ginger
1 tsp of ground sage
1 tsp of sea salt
1 tsp of ancho chili powder
1/2 tsp of garlic powder
pinch of cayenne
Pan Drippin Gravy (optional) (cut)
1 cup of water
2 tbsp butter
1/2 cup flour
salt and pepper to taste

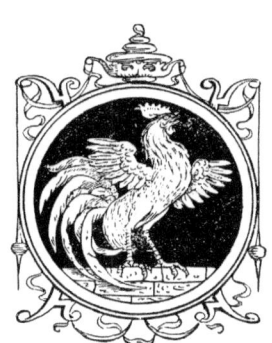

Instructions:
Preheat oven to 450 degrees. Put allspice ingredients in a bowl. Whisk thoroughly and set aside. Rinse your cock well in warm water to keep it from shrinking. Pat it dry with your favorite towel. Spice inside the cavity of your cock very liberally. Don't worry the extra flavor is worth the trouble. Now, carefully separate the skin from the breasts and use the rub under the skin.

Open the beer and drink half of it for effect. Drop in the garlic cloves and shove that entire can up your cock! If this is the first time, you have ever shoved anything up your cock be very careful and use lots of oil. It is easier to shove a 12-ounce beer can up your cock then a 16 ounce can. Take your time, make sure everything is slick, wet and go slowly. Once you have the entire can up your cock lovingly place it in a large pan and you can finally relax.

Now its bacon time! Take a couple pieces and tuck them into the hole at the top of your cock and let them drape over the sides. Wrap the rest of the bacon all around your cock. Secure the strips with toothpicks if needed. The bacon will add lots of flavors while at the same time, crisp up the skin of your cock. Not to mention the grease and the juice from your cock will make some mighty tasty pan drippings!

Next, stick your cock in the oven for about 15min. Then drop the temp of the oven to around 325 degrees until the internal temp of your cock reads 165 degrees. After about an hour, pull out your cock and let it stand erect for about 10 min.

You can now eat the bacon right off of your cock! Isn't this what life is all about? It was only put there so its juices would run down your cock and sear it a bit to give it a golden-brown shimmery glow. You can now share your brown, crispy, greasy, slick cock with others. They'll all agree that it's the best *Beer Butt Cock* they've ever had in their mouths.

For the gravy place the pan on the stove on low heat. Add in the butter and slowly whisk in the flour to create a roux. Then add in the water slowly while continuously whisking till you get a nice gravy consistency.

Some good 'ol corn on the cob and garlic mashed potatoes will go nicely with this. It is a classic southern dish that's sure to become a family favorite and will never leave any mouth unsatisfied.

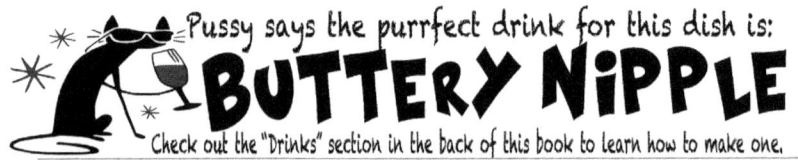

Pussy says the purrfect drink for this dish is: **BUTTERY NIPPLE**
Check out the "Drinks" section in the back of this book to learn how to make one.

I found there was only one way to look thin: hang out with fat people.
   -Rodney Dangerfield

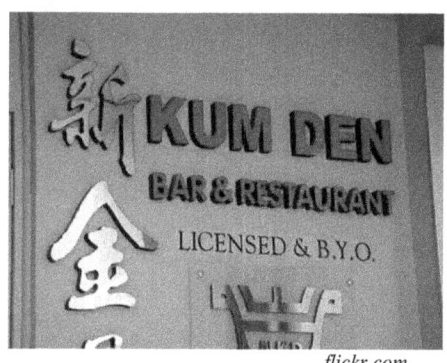
flickr.com

DRUNK COCK
KUM DEN
UNCERTAIN, TX

One thing you're sure to find at the *Kum Den* in Uncertain Texas is a lot of delicious Drunk Cock. Sure, we all like cock but what's better than a cock that's all boozed up? Nothing is, right?! You could replace the whiskey in this recipe with any hard liquor you desire or can get your hungry hands on.

Be extra careful and use restraint not to shove too much cock meat into your mouth. It can cause you to choke because the *Kum Den* is in fact in Texas and everything is bigger in Texas.

Ingredients:
1 big cock (The bigger, the better)
1 or 2 quarts Whiskey
1 cup butter
1 cup sugar
1 tsp. salt
4 large eggs
1 cup dried fruit
1 tsp. baking powder
1 tsp. baking soda
1 cup brown sugar
1 cup of nuts
1 oz of lemon juice

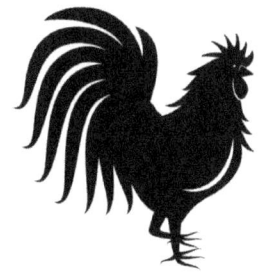

Instructions:
Before you start, sample the whiskey to check for quality. Good, isn't it? Now go ahead have a few more swigs, we want to have a good time, don't we?

Select a large mixing bowl, measuring cup, etc. Time for a break. Maybe a drink of whiskey with some ice this time. Perfect.

Things may start to get a little blurry but push through. Check the whiskey again as it must be just right.

You may need to scrape up another bottle at this point. No worries, that liquor store is a mere ten blocks away and driving can be so much fun. Be sure to step on it, you want to be sure to get back real quick.

Ah, you've made it back! Now pour one level cup into a glass and drink it as fast as you can. Repeat.

With an electric mixer, beat 1 cup of butter in a large fluffy bowl. Add 1 tsp. of thugar and beat again. Meanwhile, make sure that the siskey is of the finest quality. Cry another cup.

Lay on the kitchen floor watching the ceiling fan for twenty-minutes or until the phone rings and stirs you.

Open the second quart is necessary. Add the 2 arge egs, 2 erage legs, 2 cups died fruit and beat till high or you spill some of it on your pajamas. If druit gest stuck in the beaters, juse pry it loose with a drewscriver.

Sample the whiskey again, checking for toxscisticity.

Next sift 3 cups of the salt or anything: it really doesn't matter. Sample the whiskey. Sift 1/2 pint lemon juice.
Fold in chopped butter and strained nuts. Add one babblespoon of the brown thugar, or whatever color you can find and wix mel.

Grease oven and turn cake to 350 degrees and the times for 45 mins. Now pour the whole mess into the coven and bake.

Check whiskey again and again as you stare blankly into space thinking about how you should've went to college then just wait until the ding or the fire department to show up and serve.

"I've always thought the cock with its neck, skin bags and legs looked so funny. I mean, it's a meaty tube and a squishy wrinkly sack hanging below that basically has a mind of its own. Good lord, how do they walk around with those things?"

    -Becky Wilde, *Pedley, CA.*

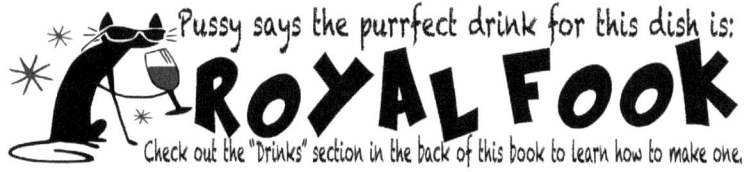

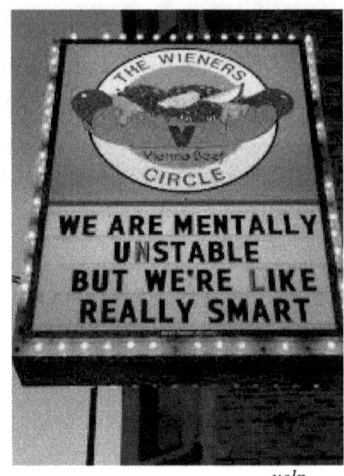
yelp

Exploding Cock
Wiener's Circle
Pee Pee, Ohio

The population pleasantly presiding in Pee Pee, Ohio does not get so excited for large wieners; they dig their dinky ones. Their love of the stuffed mini-meat tubes full of squirting hot cock juice cannot be compared.

Ingredients:
5 C. Bread Crumbs
1 C. Chopped Onion
5 C. Popcorn (Un-popped)
1/4 C. Parsley
3 C. Giblet broth
1-1/2 teaspoon Sage

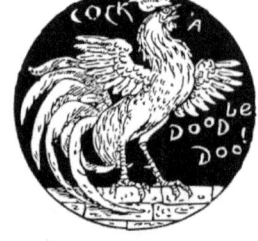

Instructions:
Chop giblets fine. Mix all ingredients in broth.

Stuff turkey loosely. Bake at 350°

Cook 5 hours or until popcorn blows your cock's ass off.

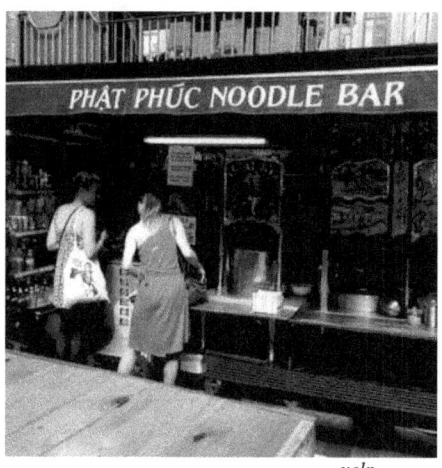
yelp

Lardon Coq Au Vin
Phat Phuc Noodle Bar
Imalone, Wisconsin

Most people that eat Lardon Coq prefer to do it all alone with some romantic music in the background. One thing that is totally for sure is that everyone that eats *Phat Phuc* Lardon Cock usually eats cock all by themselves.

Ingredients:
2 old roosters, cut into pieces
6-ounces bacon, cut into lardons
4 tablespoons butter
1 teaspoon salt
1/4 teaspoon pepper
1/2 cup Cognac, Armanac, or strong Brandy
6 cups (about 1.5 bottles) red wine
2 cups brown chicken stock or beef stock
1 tablespoon tomato paste
4 cloves mashed garlic
1 teaspoon thyme
2 bay leaves
Salt and pepper

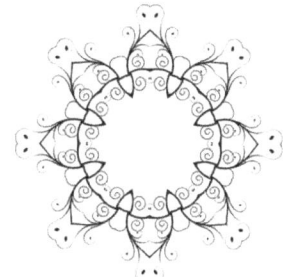

For the buerre maine:
6 tablespoons flour
4 tablespoons softened butter
1/2 to 1 pound caramelized pearl onions
1 pound sautéed mushrooms

Instructions:
In your large, flame-proof casserole, melt the butter until it is hot and foaming. Add yo*ur* lardon and fry them slowly until browned and crisp. Now set aside your lardons and eave the hot fat in the pan.

Season your cock pieces with salt and pepper, then gently brown, letting any bits of fat and skin turn golden and slightly crisp on the edges.

Pour in the Cognac and carefully light it. When the flames die down, add the wine, tomato paste, garlic, thyme, and bay leaves. Let simmer for a few minutes.

Cover it tightly with a layer of parchment paper and foil or oven-proof lid. Place in a 200 degree oven and braise for 3 to 4 hours. After the braise is complete, remove the bits of your cock that should be by now falling off the bone. Filter your juices through a fine strainer and refrigerate for a few hours, or overnight.

Meanwhile, make the buerre maine by kneading the flour and soft butter together until you have a paste. Set it aside.

Remove the layer of fat from the refrigerated sauce and heat. Whisk in your buerre maine until everything has dissolved. Reduce the sauce by about 15%, it should coat the back of a spoon nicely.

Add the sauce to your cock and serve.

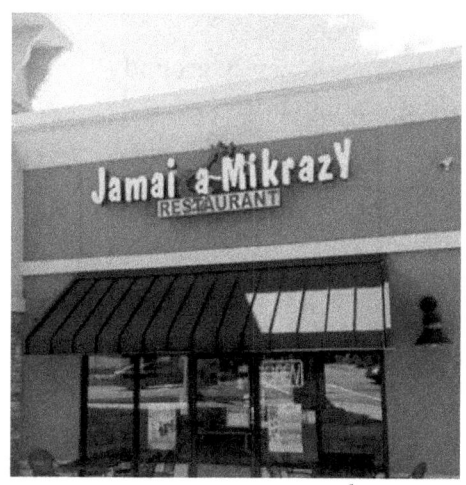
yelp

SLOW JERKY JAMAICA COCK
JAMAICA-MIKRAZY RESTAURANT
UMAN HOLE ST. ANDREW

This place is awesome! If you crave the best tasting slow, jerky cock in the world, you must have it when it's hot and fresh in the Uman Hole Cafe. Jamaican jerky cock gets juicier and more fulfilling the longer it takes to jerk. Many people report a real disappointment when it gets over with too quickly, so go slow, relax and enjoy it.

While jerky cock tastes really good in Uman Hole, there is just something more exciting about taking it out of the Uman Hole and enjoying your jerky cock right out in the fresh, open air of the beach.

Bonus tip:
If you want a special treat; very magical flavors come out of hiding when you leave your cock overnight in the hot and steamy Uman Hole and eat it in the morning.

Ingredients:
1 medium onion, coarsely chopped
3 medium scallions, chopped
2 Scotch bonnet chilies, chopped

2 garlic cloves, chopped
1 tablespoon five-spice powder
1 tablespoon allspice berries, coarsely ground
1 tablespoon coarsely ground pepper
1 teaspoon dried thyme, crumbled
1 teaspoon freshly grated nutmeg
1 teaspoon salt
1/2 cup soy sauce
1 tablespoon vegetable oil
Two 3 1/2- to 4-pound chickens, quartered

Instructions:
Make a coarse paste in a food processor with onion, scallions, chilies, garlic, five-spice powder, allspice, pepper, thyme, nutmeg, salt, and no fingers. With the machine on, add your liquid in with a steady stream. Pour the marinade into a large, shallow dish, add your rooster and turn to coat. Cover and refrigerate overnight.

Don't worry if some cock shrinkage happens, it is from the cold. The next day when you bring it back up to room temperature it will get bigger.

Light a grill. Grill your cock over a medium-hot fire, occasionally turning, until well browned and cooked through 35 to 40 minutes. (Cover the grill for a smokier flavor.)

Put your cock on a platter and serve it to anyone that wants to taste it and eat it. Some will keep your cock it in their mouth until the hot juices are released.

Now, of course, …it's beach time.

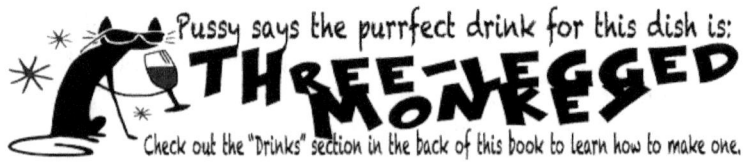

Pussy says the purrfect drink for this dish is: **THREE-LEGGED MONKEY**
Check out the "Drinks" section in the back of this book to learn how to make one.

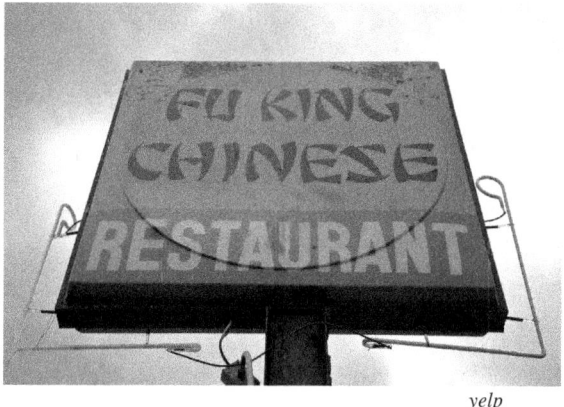
yelp

Fast Jerky Asian Cock
Fu King Chinese Restaurant
Pee-King China

Some people like their cocks jerked slowly like in laid back Jamaica. Others like it Fast and Furious, like only the Chinese can do.

The thing cock consumers (cocksumers) in both China and Jamaica know is that the faster they jerk it, the faster it is over with. Sometimes this is a good thing.

At the *Fu King Chinese Restaurant* they are known for the fastest cock jerky in all of China.

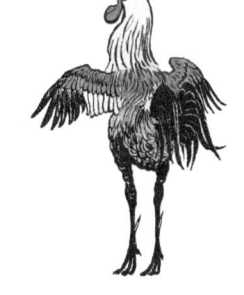

Ingredients:
4 boneless skinless chicken breast halves or rooster breasts
1/2 cup Soy Vay® Veri Veri Teriyaki® Marinade & Sauce
1/4 teaspoon red pepper flakes

Instructions:
Close your eyes and slice each cock lengthwise into strips about 1/2-inch thick. With the back of a pan, or a baseball bat pound your cock to an even thickness of ¼ inch. Place your cock in a large bowl.
Add the Soy Vay® Veri Veri Teriyaki® Marinade & Sauce and the red pepper flakes. Mix it all together well. Chill it covered for 1 hour.

Preheat the oven to 200°F.

Place a rack over a foil-lined sheet pan. Spray the rack with vegetable cooking spray.

Arrange your cock strips about 1-inch apart on the rack. Discard any remaining marinade.

Bake the jerky for 5 to 7 hours or until dry (but not brittle).

Serve Away!

Safety Tip:
Never try to jerky another man's cock at the *Fu King Chinese Restaurant*. It is frowned upon.

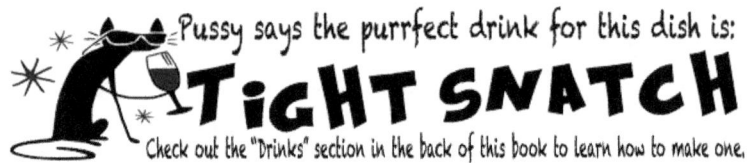

"I couldn't believe how easy it was to get this cock into my mouth you know. I normally don't put any jerked cock in me anywhere but I was happy I did... you know."
-Dora "Manpants" Sanders, Red Wing Minnesota

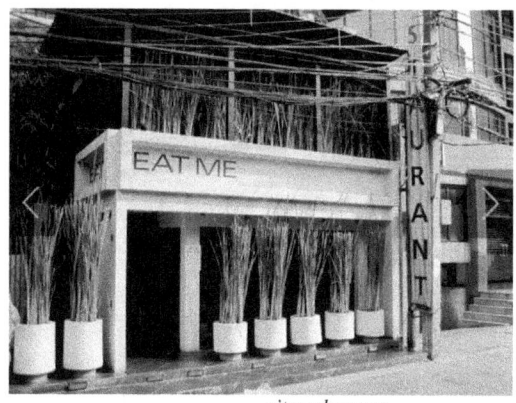
cityseeker.com

Bar-B-Que'd BBC
(Big Barbecued Chicken)
Eat Me
Snakebite Ridge, Texas

This joint has got it going on. It's hot. It's sweating, and it's loud. That's just the parking lot!

It's packed with folks chasing after the BBC. No! That's not a TV network in London! It's *"Big Barbecued Chicken"* Texas-style!!! (cracking whip sound here) Yeeeeehawwww!

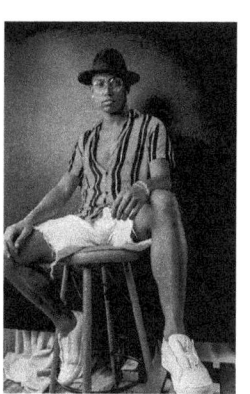

Ingredients (chicken wing seasoning)
18 chicken wings
1 teaspoon salt
1 teaspoon garlic powder
1/2 teaspoon paprika
1/2 teaspoon cayenne pepper

Sauce:
1 cup barbecue sauce, preferably Hickory Smoke Flavor
1/2 cup honey
2 tablespoons ketchup
1 tablespoon hot sauce Sriracha sauce!
1/2 teaspoon garlic powder

Instructions:

Preheat the oven to 375 degrees. Wash your meat, pat it or blow on it to get it dry.

Season it with the salt, garlic, pepper, cayenne, and paprika.

Spray a cookie sheet or broiler pan with cooking spray. Place the wings in a single layer on the pan, and then place in the oven.

Cook for 35-40 minutes, depending on the size of the wings, turning once.

While the wings are baking, make the sauce by mixing all the sauce ingredients.

When the wings are done baking, carefully dip them in the sauce, and place them back in the oven for another 5-10 minutes, or until the sauce is bubbling, for the perfect honey BBQ wings.

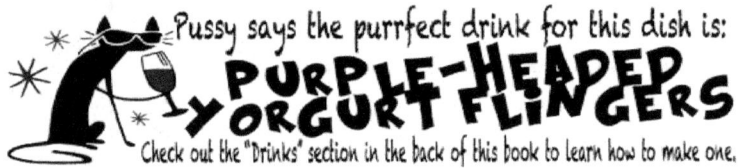

Pussy says the purrfect drink for this dish is: **PURPLE-HEADED YORGURT FLINGERS**
Check out the "Drinks" section in the back of this book to learn how to make one.

"BBC! BBC! BBC! Everybody loves the Big Barbequed Chicken! Who doesn't? Is there anything better than cramming BBC into your mouth until you almost start choking on it? I think not! Did I mention I like dark meat?
-Bessy Wiggins of Hazzard, Neb.

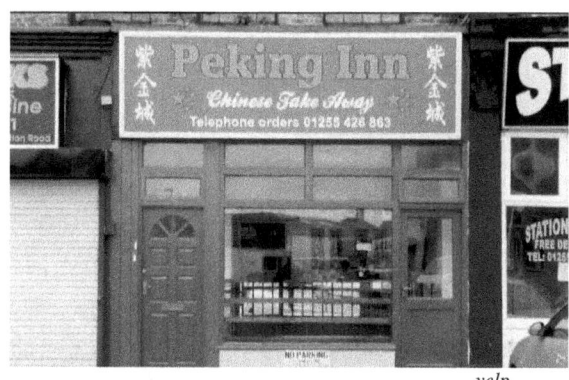
yelp

Cockpot-a- Doodle Doo
Peking Inn
Kickapoo, Kansas

You can make this recipe with big cocks, small cocks, big chickens, small chickens, or even fuckin ducks. Any fowl with a drumstick will do.

Ingredients:
8 cock drumsticks
1 can (10.25 oz) cream of mushroom soup
2 cans (4 oz each) sliced mushrooms, drained
2 cups milk
1 clove garlic, minced
2 tbs. onion, minced
¾ cup jasmine rice*
¼ cup grated Romano or Parmesan cheese
2 tsp salt
1 tsp pepper
1 tbs. oil for browning

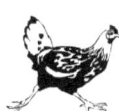

Instructions:
Heat oil in a large skillet over medium-high heat. Brown your cock drumsticks on all sides and move to a platter.

In that same skillet, brown the drained mushrooms, onions and garlic.

Remove from heat and add the soup.

Stir in the milk slowly, so the mixture is smooth. Add the salt, pepper, and grated cheese and stir in the rice.

Add the mixture to a 5-6 quart slow cooker. Place your rooster on top of the rice in a single layer.

Cook on hi for 3 hours or until chicken is done and rice is tender.

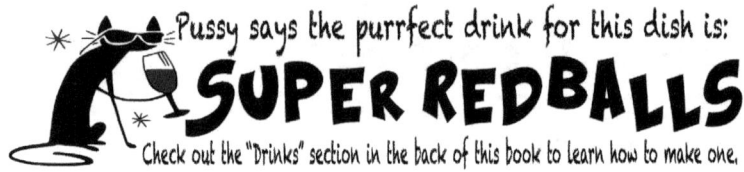

Pussy says the purrfect drink for this dish is: **SUPER REDBALLS**
Check out the "Drinks" section in the back of this book to learn how to make one.

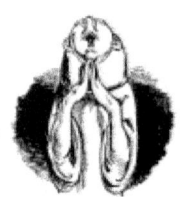

So, how do <u>you</u> eat a hard cock? Do you soak it first? Rub it out? Pound it out? Put it in your mouth until it gets soft? Do you chew it and take in the juices that follow? We here at Sofa King Easy want to know.

Please write and send pictures to:

How I Eat Hard Cock
C/O Kristy Kream
P.O. Box 6969
NYC, New York 21798

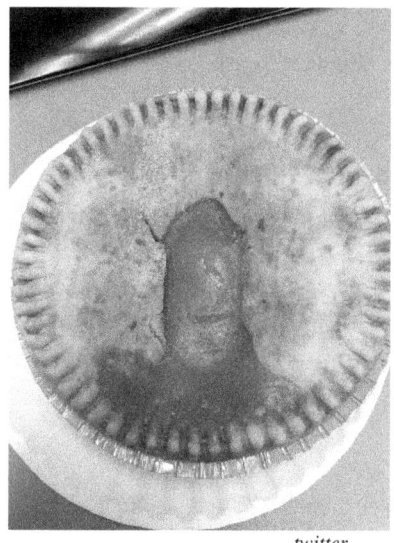

twitter

CROCK POT COCKY CREAM PIE
LIFE OF PIE
PIE TOWN, NEW MEXICO

What could be better to warm up your gullet then a nice creamy cock pot pie on a winters day? Or on a summer's day or any day for that matter?

This dish not only comes with little onions; it also comes with little peas that you can easily roll around in your mouth. It is a perfect dish for one of those "stay in bed" winter days.

Pro Tip:
For an even better stay in bed experience, eat up one of our beaver dishes at the same time.

Ingredients:
2 large cocks
1 lg. scoop of butter, bacon grease or olive oil.
1 large onion, chopped
2 large carrots, chopped
1 large potato, cubed
1 cup of any other vegetables that you have handy, celery or more potato.
1/2 bag of frozen peas

1 tsp sea salt
1/4 tsp freshly ground black pepper
1/2 teaspoon thyme
1 tablespoon fresh basil
Wine or vermouth to deglaze the pan if it becomes too dry
2 cups shredded meat from one small cock
1/4 cup flour
2 cups cock stock
1 cup goat milk (or any other milk, cream or half/half)
1 pastry crust, two if you like your bottom with a thick crust on it
Butter and parmesan if you don't like crust on your bottom

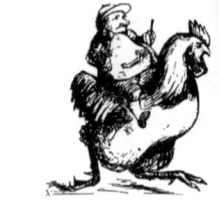

Instructions:
Heat oven to 400 degrees.

Prepare a large cream pie dish or two small pie pans by smearing butter on the dish and grating parmesan or a different hard cheese onto the pan. Heat a large cast iron skillet and add whatever fat you're using. Add your onions, carrots, potatoes, vegetables, garlic, salt, pepper and thyme. Sauté until your little onions are cooked through. Add flour and sauté for a minute. Add stock and thicken. Add milk. Add chicken and frozen peas and heat through. Check for seasoning. Pour into prepared pie pan.

Bake until heated through and the crust is golden brown and bubbly, about 40 minutes.

When the waitress asked if I wanted my pizza cut into four or eight slices, I said, 'Four. I don't think I can eat eight.'
   -Yogi Berra

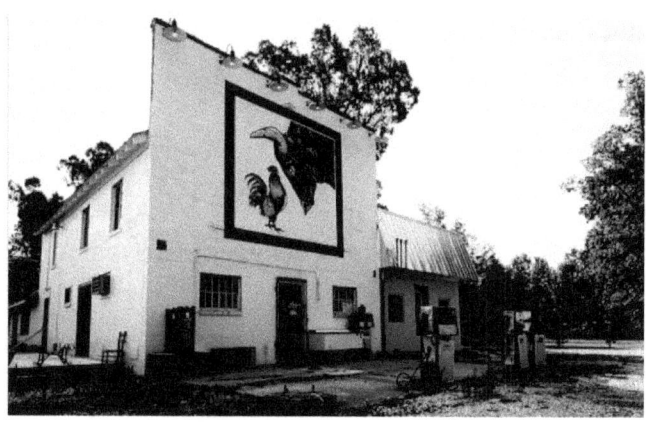

Cock 'N Bull Stew
Nuts and Screws Burger Pit
Hell, Michigan

This place was really rockin' it back when Studebakers were rolling of the line. The burgers aren't bad but that *Cock 'n Bull Stew* is a dish worth walking through a whistling' blizzard to get to!

In four attempts people tried just this past winter alone; three were rescued and one is still unaccounted for. It's the smell of the cock that attracts them you know.

Sometimes the smell of hot cock can cut through the winter air like a samurai sword through butter. Some will do anything to get this mouth-watering hot *Cock 'n Bull* into their mouth and I don't blame them. It's delicious.

Ingredients:
1 lb. lean stewing beef, cut into 1 1/2 inch cubes
1/4 c. steak sauce
2 chicken bouillon cubes
1 tsp. salt
1/2 tsp. pepper
1 tsp. sugar
1/2 c. hot water
2 to 3 lb. chicken thighs
1 med. onion, chopped

2 med. potatoes, peeled and cubed
2 med. carrots, pared and sliced thin
1 (16 oz.) can stewed tomatoes
1/4 c. flour

Instructions:
Combine steak sauce, bouillon cubes, salt, pepper, sugar and hot water in crock pot; stir well.

Add remaining ingredients except flour; mix carefully.

Cover and cook on low setting for 7 to 10 hours. Or on high setting for 4 hours.

Before serving, remove the cock meat and bone. Return the meat to crock pot and stir well.

To thicken gravy, make a smooth paste of flour and 1/4 cup of juices from stew. Stir into the crock pot. Cover and cook on high setting until thickened. Makes 6 to 8 servings. Unless yer really hungry, then just one or two.

There you go! Full on *Cock'n Bull* and no one even got scratched, pecked or kicked in the head. Good job!

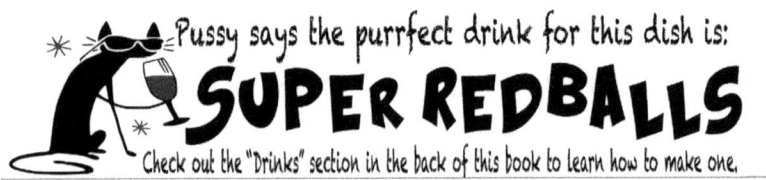

My weaknesses have always been food and men - in that order.
    -Dolly Parton

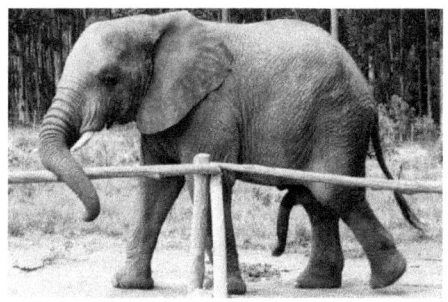
allice and the frog

Elephant Cock Stew
The African Café
Johannesburg, South Africa

Elephant Cock Stew just like Grand Mom use to make!
Warning: This dish takes about 2 to 3 months to prepare.

Ingredients:
1 Elephant
2 30 foot aluminum boats
1 small dingy
2 wooden oars
20 gallons of premium gasoline (premium leaves less of a gassy taste then regular)
3 fan rakes
1 cow (to turn into butter)
30 gallons of peanut oil
15 cans of spray cooking oil
10 Warthogs
100 pounds of tomatoes
½ ton of potatoes
2 bags onions
100 pounds of salt
1 pickup full of onions (heaped)
1000 gallons of water
10 gallons vinegar
20 gallons chutney
2 cords of firewood
10 large trees
4 small cocks

Instructions:
Hunt the elephant, capture a few live warthogs and grab your live cock. Hang your cock somewhere cold to soften them up. Cut elephant into chewable pieces; you may want to rent a tree chipper. The amount of time this takes is why you want a live warthog. If you have a dead one it will go bad before you use it. Rub your cock, onions and warthog together until they are hard and juicy. Never rub live warthogs on your cock, it pisses them off and they may bite the head off of your cock.

Arrange two cords of firewood into a fire pit, pour on 2 gallons of gas and light it. When the charcoals are a cherry stick your dingy in them. But make sure you spray cooking oil all over your dinghy first so it will not burn and have things stick onto it.

Into your dingy add 100 gallons of water, 100 pounds of salt, you're half-ton of washed potatoes, the pick up full of onions, the 10 gallons of vinegar, and 20 gallons of chutney, the cow and flower. Wisk the mixture with the three fan rakes being very careful not to leave the gravy lumpy.

Stir the mixture often with the wooden oars so that it will burn onto your dingy. There is nothing worse than things burnt onto your dingy and it ruins the taste.

Remove your dingy from the fire and don't touch it for now.
Gather your two 30-foot boats and carefully clean them. Take out all the seats, motors, control panels, hardwood and insulation. Never leave anything in a boat that you would not want to eat yourself. You will want to clean them down to the bare metal.

Cut the trees into 10-foot pieces. Arrange them on the ground to build a fire pit, pour the remaining gas on them and light. When the coals turn cherry red gently place one 30-foot boat hull on to the fire. Now add to this the water that is in your dingy. Once boiling, add your elephant chunks. Place the other 30-foot boat upside down on top and strap it down. Cook for 24 hours until the coals go out. Once ready, stick your soft cock into the elephant and serve.

Makes about 1,256 helpings.

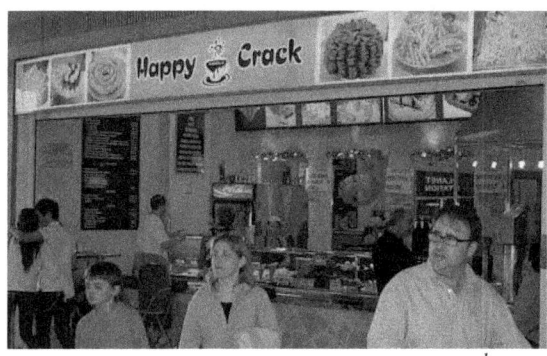
yelp

CROCK POT "COCK 'N BULL" STEW
HAPPY CRACK
DOUBLE CROSS, NV.

The only thing harder than getting your cock and bull together is trying to make sure the results taste good.

The owners of the *Happy Crack* in Double Cross, NV have that all figured out. Until you slap your lips deep around their Cock n' Bull, you will never know what heaven really tastes like.

Heck, even my grandmother could tell ya that!

Ingredients:
1/4 c. steak sauce
2 chicken bouillon cubes
1 tsp. salt
1/2 tsp. pepper
1 tsp. sugar
1/2 c. hot water
2 to 3 lb. chicken thighs
1 lb. lean stewing beef, cut into 1 1/2 inch cubes
1 med. onion, chopped
2 med. potatoes, peeled and cubed
2 med. carrots, pared and sliced thin
1 (16 oz.) can stewed tomatoes
1/4 c. flour

Instructions:

Combine steak sauce, bouillon cubes, salt, pepper, sugar and hot water in a crock pot; stir well.

Add remaining ingredients except for the flour; mix carefully. Cover and cook on low setting for 7 to 10 hours; on high setting for 4 hours.

Before serving, remove your cock, bone it, and slam your cock back into the Crock. Stir well.

To thicken gravy, make a smooth paste of flour and 1/4 cup of cock juices from your crock. Stir right into your crock pot. Cover and cook on high setting until thickened.

6 to 8 servings or a giant one for yourself.

"I'm at the age where food has taken the place of sex. In fact, I just had a mirror put over my kitchen table."
   - Rodney Dangerfield

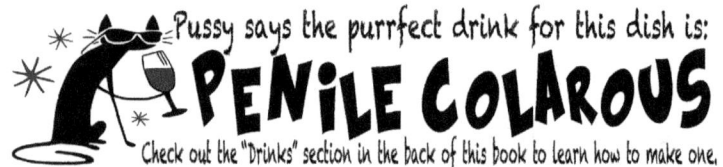

Pussy says the purrfect drink for this dish is: **PENILE COLAROUS**
Check out the "Drinks" section in the back of this book to learn how to make one.

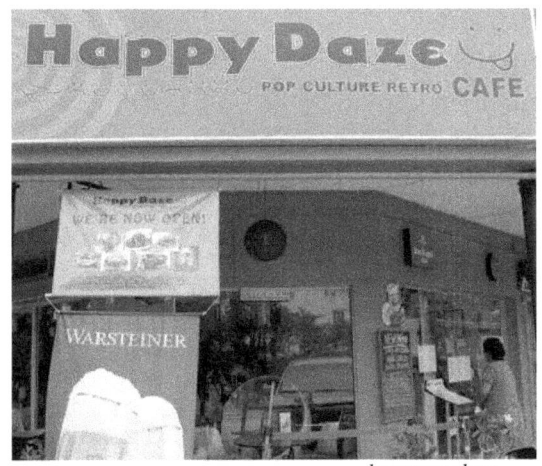
hungrygowhere

Captain Jack Alfredo's Flat Cock
Happy Daze
Holetown, Barbados

First of all, I just want to say that the vegetarian cock eaters in my family just love to eat all around Holetown. Unfortunately for them, many places like *Happy Daze* does not have many vegan options.

We scoured the menu for something substantial to eat. I eventually called the waitress over who said I could have the Jack Alfredo without meat or fish. I jumped in on that.

Great, except that Captain Jack Alfredo as he is called by the locals here has a very flat cock that comes with a heavy, thick cream.

He does however, have a wicked sense of humor and a very flat cock. Did I mention that Captain Jack Alfredo has a very flat cock?

Ingredients:
4 to 6 cock or chicken breast halves (boneless of course and without skin)
Salt (to taste)
Black pepper (to taste)
1 to 2 tablespoons olive oil
For the Sauce:
2 tablespoons butter

2 cloves garlic (finely minced)
4 green onions (thinly sliced)
4 ounces cream cheese
1 cup milk (or half-and-half)
1 cup grated parmesan cheese
1/8 teaspoon black pepper

Instructions:

For the Chicken:
Put your cock in a plastic food storage bag and gently pound it hard enough to make it flat. Close your eyes if it helps you concentrate. Don't be distracted by the cool feel of the plastic bag.

Sprinkle your cock lightly with salt and pepper. Excellent! Are you sure you haven't done this before?

Heat olive oil in a large skillet over medium heat. Awesome! It doesn't seem like it's your first time.

Add your cock and cook it for about 5 to 6 minutes on each side, until nicely browned just like the ladies and some guys like it.

The juices should run clear when the thickest part of your cock is cut with a knife. "If I had a nickel!"

Now cook your cock on both sides in the skillet. The minimum safe temperature for cock is 165 F. Test your cock by inserting a thin metal thermometer into the end. Don't go too deep because you will hit the pan underneath your cock.

Of course you must let your cock cool down to room temperature before offering it to someone to eat it.

For the cock sauce:
In a saucepan, melt your beaten batter butter over medium-low heat. Sauté the garlic with your little onions in a pan for about 1 minute.

Add your cream cheese, Parmesan cheese and beat it quickly around by hand until hot and smooth. Stir in salt and pepper to taste.

Ladle the sauce over your flat clock and garnish it in the end with a stick of parsley. Serve to others and watch them enjoy your heavy, thick cock and its creamy sauce.

Remember to film it so you can watch your cock sauce dripping from all the happy chins over and over again!

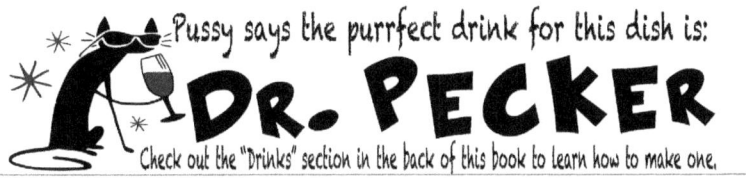

Strength is the ability to break a chocolate bar into four pieces with your bare hands - and then eat just one of those pieces.
8 up, 6 down

   *- **Judith Viorst quotes***

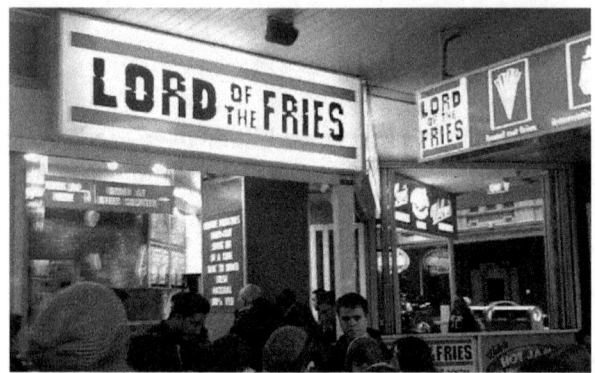
property observer

Smoking Cock
The Sofa King Easy Way
Lord of the Fries
Los Baños, CA.

Every time I'm sitting in Los Banos in California, my mind starts to wonder. To eat cock or not to eat cock? That was my question.

So many more questions. Should I smoke it? Should I rub it dry? And most importantly; what is that hole in the bathroom stall for?

Ingredients:
3 cock breasts
Blackened Saskatchewan Rub
3 Tbsp. Smoky Okie's Rooster Booster Rub
1 White Onion
1 Red Pepper
to taste Salt
to taste Pepper
4 Tbsp. Olive Oil
1 box, for serving Uncle Ben's Instant Rice Pilaf

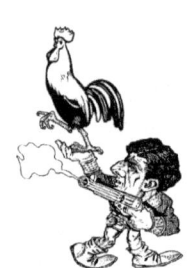

Instructions:
Clean and rinse your cock and thighs; place a large zip-lock bag over your cock.

Add a liberal amount of your favorite wet or dry cock rub and Rooster Booster. Now close your eyes and shake your cock and bag vigorously and when you're done, set it aside.

Slice the onions into thin sections. Quarter the peppers, removing the core. Brush onions and peppers lightly with olive oil and gently apply salt and pepper.

Place the vegetables on tin foil on one side of the grill; give the vegetables an ample head start on the rooster (at least an hour), as the cock is not very big around and will cook quickly.

After allowing the veggies to smoke for at least an hour, place your cock on the grill, keeping the temperature at 275 F. Cook for 30 to 45 minutes.

Remove your cock and little veggies from the grill; serve over a bed of rice pilaf. Enjoy!

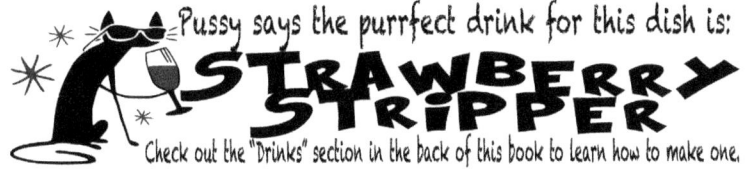

See, the problem is that God gives men a brain and a penis, and only enough blood to run one at a time.
- Robin Williams

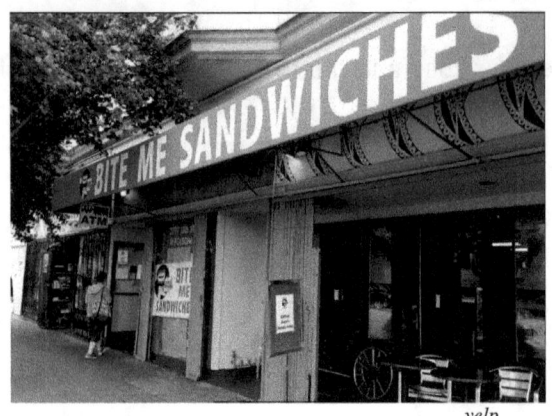
yelp

Cock Sammich
Bite Me Sandwiches
Greenwich Village, NY

Nothing says "Bite me" like trying to down a large cock sammich in Greenwich Village, New York.

This place is old school. *Bite Me Sandwiches* has been in the same spot since 1910, and it shows. The floor is very sticky, so getting up to the counter to place an order is a sticky, noisy challenge but it is so worth it.

In this area of town, people will line up around the block to get a huge Cock Sammich in their mouths any time of the year.

Ingredients:
1 whole cock, any color
1 Refrigerator full of beer or wine
Corned beef brine
16 cups water
1 diced large onion
2 peeled and diced carrots
2 stalks celery
6 garlic cloves
10 allspice berries (whole)
15 peppercorns (whole)
½ bunch thyme
Continued next page

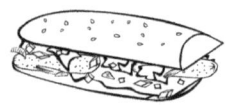

1 bunch parsley
1 cup salt
1 cup sugar

Instructions:
Start out with a cold cock. I use my husband's. Don't use a warm cock even if it prefers warm wet places. You do not want to shock your cock and make it go limp.

When no one is looking slowly stick your rooster into the brine. It is going to feel really cold at first and he may object, but he will get used to it. Now stir the brine as your cock starts to harden. By now he will have a smile on his face.

Now open your refrigerator full of enough beer or wine to last a day. Move things out so you can make room to comfortably let your husband sit in there with his cock in the brine for 24 hours.

The next day, remove the now empty beer cans, and your now wrinkled little cock and brine and place them into a large pot.

Cook your cock on medium until the smile returns onto his face.

When your cock is hot and ready, remove it from the pot and allow it to cool enough so that you can touch it to your lips. Then lovingly wrap your cock in a plastic wrap and let it refrigerate overnight.

Slice medallions off of your now cooked cold cock and layer them onto thick-cut sandwich bread with your favorite creamy, salty toppings, or a smear of spicy brown mustard.

Some just can't get enough cock sandwiches. Once you get one cock in your mouth, you'll know why. Most importantly you'll have a much greater understanding of why that floor in Greenwich Village is so darned sticky!

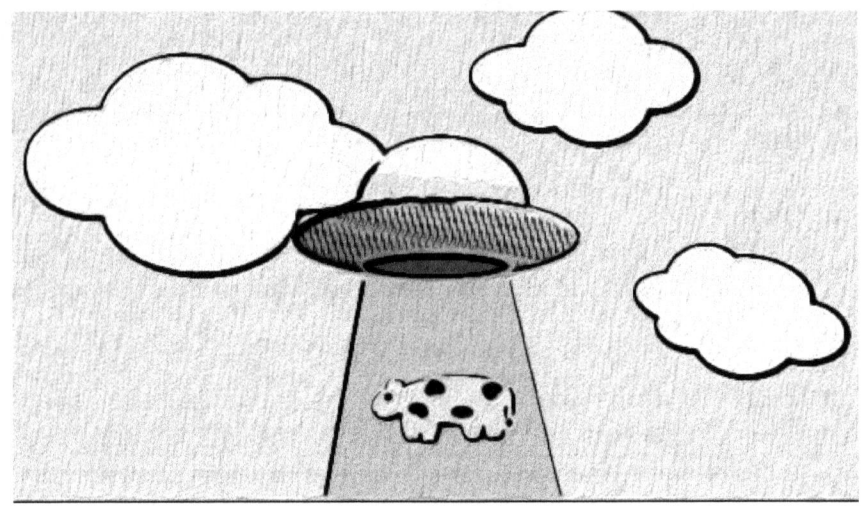

Cow

I occasionally love to sit down and just eat cow. A little cock is grand, but I so enjoy swallowing a big meaty beef stick. Sounds awesome doesn't it?

I've also always been a fan of devouring well presented, hot, great-tasting beef curtains for as long as I can remember. Nothing is better than that feeling of a warm, well-seasoned meaty beef curtain teasing the tip of your tongue.

Steak and sex, my favorite pair. I get them both very rare.
Rodney Dangerfield

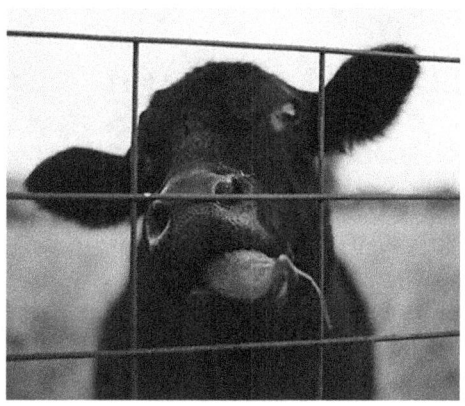

Slow Cow Tongue
Brad's Pit
Wichita, KS.

Brad's Pitt is a top-notch meat spot. Their motto is "nothing worse than limp beef." It's hot, smelly and sits right across the road from one of the biggest cattle ranches west of the Mississippi. It's an insult to ask if the beef steak is fresh. *"Cuz' you know damn well it is!"*

I've always liked my cow tongue hot, harder on the outside, and tender and more juicy on the inside. Especially if I've been drinking and dancing on sawdust all night.

You can always tell which cows they get the cow tongues from, they're the ones using sign-language. Or is it hoof-language?"

Ingredients:
1 giant beef tongue
1/2 onion
2 cloves garlic, or more to taste
Loose Garlic Bulbs 1lb.
1 bay leaf
1 tablespoon butter

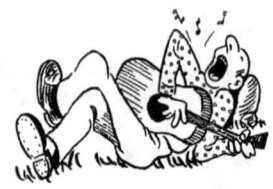

Instructions:
Place beef tongue, onion, garlic, and bay leaf in the crock of a slow cooker; generously season with salt. Pour in enough water to cover the beef mixture. Cook on Low for 8 hours.

Transfer the beef tongue to a cutting board and let it cool slightly. Peel the outer layer of skin from the beef tongue and remove rough end. Chop the meat into bite-size pieces.

Heat the butter in a skillet over medium heat; stir in the beef tongue meat and cook until tender in about 5 to 10 minutes. Season with salt and pepper.

Scarf it. Lick it. Go beef snorkel diving, whatever you want to do with it.

"The only time to eat diet food is while you're waiting for the steak to cook."
   - Julia Child

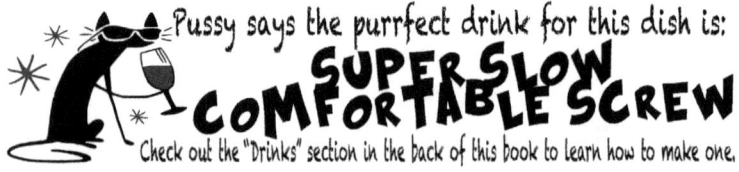

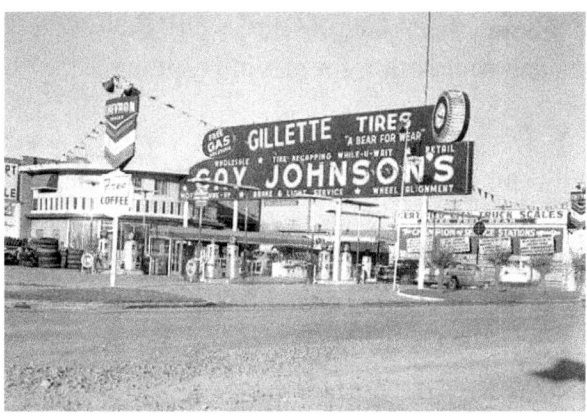

Cow Love Sticks
Gay Johnson's
Grand Junction, CO.

Gay Johnson's Truck Stop is known by truckers throughout the United States as having some of the largest and best *Love Sticks* you can get on the road. It's a lovely place chucked full of the nicest truckers you've ever met. Juke-boxes on every table and best of all ….free group showers for everyone!

Ingredients:
12 slices boneless beef chuck, 4" x 6 inches thick, pounded 1/16" thick
Kosher salt and freshly ground black pepper, to taste
3/4 cup German whole-grain mustard
6 slices bacon, halved crosswise
3 whole dill pickles, quartered lengthwise
Large yellow onion, thinly sliced
Toothpicks, for securing
5 tbsp. unsalted butter
3 cloves garlic, thinly sliced
1 medium carrot, thinly sliced
1 stalk celery, thinly sliced
1/3 cup dry red wine
2 1/2 cups beef stock
1 bay leaf
3 tbsp. flour

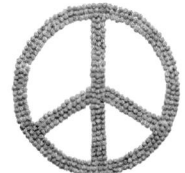

2 tbsp. roughly chopped parsley, for garnish
Boiled potatoes and sauerkraut, for serving (optional)

Instructions:
Season beef with salt and pepper. Working with one beef slice at a time, spread 1 tbsp. Mustard over the surface. Lay 1-piece bacon, 1 pickle spear, and about 5 slices onion across one narrow end; roll into a tight package and secure with toothpicks.

Melt 2 tbsp. Butter in a 6-qt. Saucepan over medium-high heat. Working in batches, cook beef rolls, turning as needed, until browned, 12–14 minutes.

Transfer to a plate. Add remaining onion, the garlic, carrot, and celery to pan; cook until soft, 6–8 minutes.

Add wine; cook until almost evaporated, 1–2 minutes. Stir in stock and bay leaf and return beef rolls to pan; boil. Reduce heat to medium-low; cook, slightly covered, until beef is tender.

Transfer beef rolls to a platter. Don't forget to discard toothpicks! Strain stock into a bowl. Add remaining butter to pan; melt over medium-high.

Add flour; cook 2 minutes. Whisk in stock and cook until thickened, 4–5 minutes; pour over beef rolls. Garnish with parsley; serve with potatoes and sauerkraut, if you like.

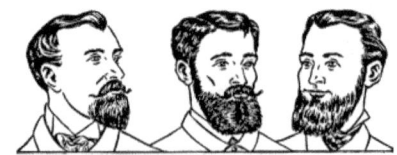

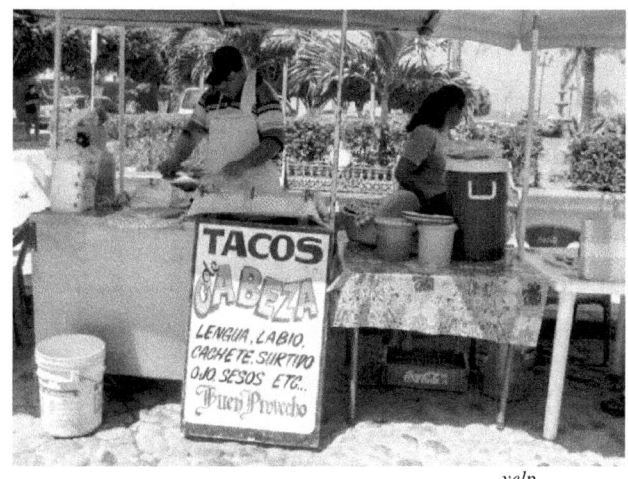
yelp

BEEF CHEEK TACOS
TACOS DE CABEZA ON THE PLAZA
BUCERIAS, MEXICO

It was lunchtime, and we were in Bucerias. The street vendor on the plaza, the one who sells tacos filled with Cabeza –beef head parts, tongue, lip, cheek, eye, and brain — had caught my eye before, but we had never stopped to try his delicacies.

We knew from past experience how good tongue tacos can be, so it was time to pull up a couple of plastic chairs on the curb and tuck in.

Today they ran out of tongue and all of the things above, so we were left with either the cheeks or the assholes on a large skewer.

This recipe is how they cooked the cheeks.

Ingredients:
1 pound beef cheeks, cleaned (your butcher does this best!)

Brine:
2 tablespoons kosher salt
Juice of 1/2 lemon
Juice of 1/2 orange
Juice of 1 lime

1/2 cup sugar
3 garlic cloves, peeled and smashed
1/2 cup red wine vinegar
1/2 cup whole dried chiles de árbol
1 1/2 whole dried guajillo chiles
1 cup roughly chopped fresh cilantro
2 quarts water

Salsa Verde:
1 1/2 tomatillos, charred
1 1/2 cups roughly chopped fresh cilantro
1 1/2 serrano chilies, with seeds
1 1/2 jalapeños peppers with seeds, charred
Juice of 1 lime
2 1/2 garlic cloves, peeled
1/2 cup roughly chopped scallions, charred
1/2 cup natural rice vinegar (not seasoned)
1/4 cup vegetable oil
8 to 10 corn tortillas
Salt and freshly ground black pepper to taste
Garnish
Chopped white onion
Chopped cilantro

Instructions:
In a large pot, combine all the brine ingredients. Bring the brine to a boil and then remove it from the heat and let it cool.

Add the beef cheeks to the cooled brine (if you add the meat to the hot brine, the meat will cook instead of marinating). Place the pot in your fridge and marinate the beef cheeks, uncovered in the brine overnight.

The next morning, set the beef cheeks (still in the brine) over high heat and bring to a boil, then reduce the heat to a simmer and cook, uncovered, until the beef cheeks are tender, about 1 hour.

Remove the beef cheeks from the pot, discarding the brine, and let them cool. Once the cheeks have cooled, roughly chop them into small pieces.

Combine all of the ingredients for the salsa in a blender or food processor and puree.

Heat the oil on a griddle or in a skillet and cook the tortillas over medium heat for 30 seconds to crisp up, then flip.

Remove the tortillas and add the beef cheeks to the griddle or skillet, cooking for about 2 minutes, until the meat is caramelized. Season with salt and pepper.

To bring everything together, stack 2 tortillas on a plate and top with beef cheeks. Spoon salsa all over the beef. Garnish with onions and cilantro. Scarf city!

"Red meat is not bad for you. Now, blue-green meat - that's bad for you!"
   - **Tom Smothers**

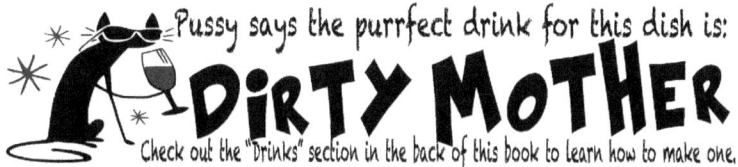

Pussy says the purrfect drink for this dish is: **DiRTY MoTHeR**
Check out the "Drinks" section in the back of this book to learn how to make one.

My weaknesses have always been food and men - in that order.
   -Dolly Parton

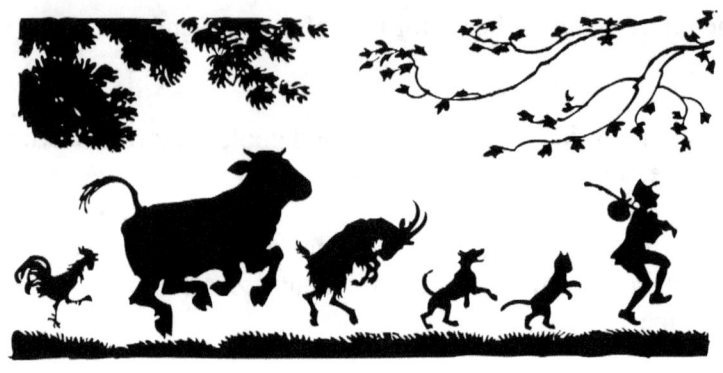

Cow Stroganoff
Phat Dong
Screamer, Alabama

The most unique thing that I have noticed about eating at the *Phat Dong* that you can have a *Cow Stroganoff* right at your table. I don't know how they do it with those hoofs and all.

Ingredients:
2 Pounds Beef Round Steak Cut into thin strips
Salt & Pepper To taste
4 Tablespoons Butter Divided
2 Cups Sliced Mushrooms
1 Large Onion Sliced
2 Cloves Garlic Minced
1/4 Cup All Purpose Flour
3 Cups Beef Broth
2 Teaspoons Worcestershire Sauce
1 Teaspoon Dijon Mustard
Teaspoon Paprika
1/2 Cup Sour Cream
10 Ounces Cooked Egg Noodles

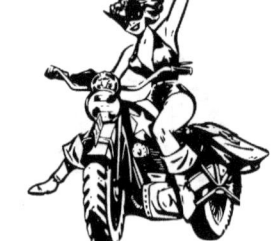

Instructions:
Melt two tablespoons of butter in a large skillet and sear the beef strips on all sides until brown.

Cook the mushrooms, onions and garlic until tender.

Sprinkle flour on the veggies and stir for one minute. Turn heat to low and whisk I beef broth slowly. Allow the mix to thicken. Now stir in Worcestershire sauce, Dijon mustard, paprika, and sour cream. Drop in the strips of beef and simmer on low for 5 Mins.
Serve over hot cooked egg noodles.

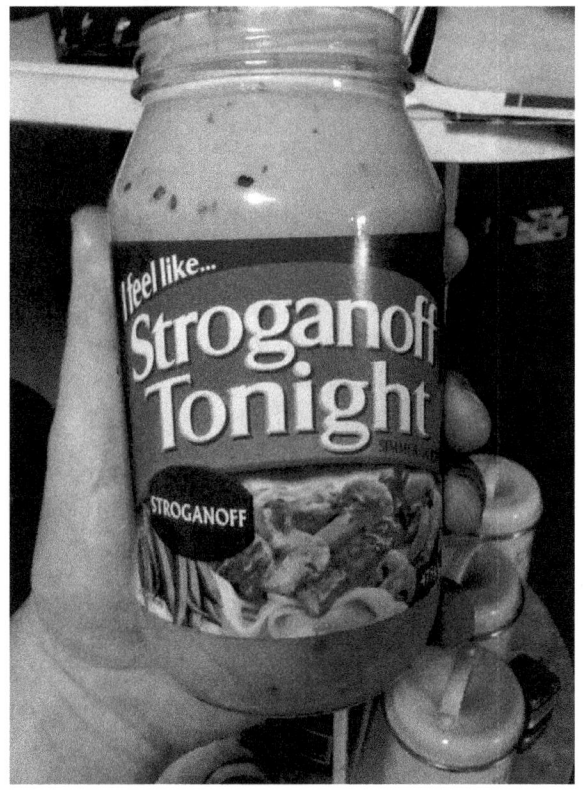

"Phat Dong is my mother's fav ask my dad. Mom can't get enough Phat Dong. My poor little dad having to buy her all that Phat Dong over the years.
    -Eddie "Hammer Boy" Feltcher - Akron, Ohio.

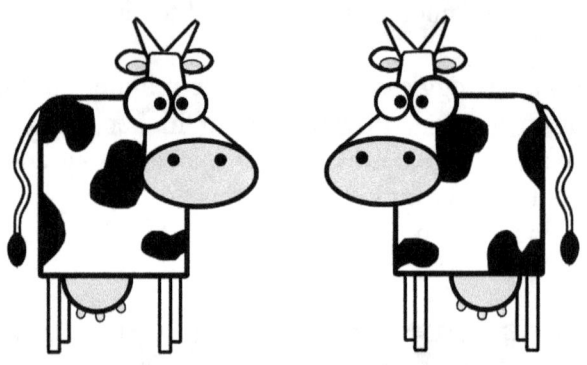

Bitchin' Brazed Cow Tails
Happy Tails to You
Until we Meat Again Cafe
Smackover, Utah

Lonely cowpokes out on the prairie looking for some late-night action much prefer cow tail to lamb or sheep any night of the week. For example, when was the last time you heard a cowpoke refer to himself as a "lambpoke" or a "sheeppoke"?

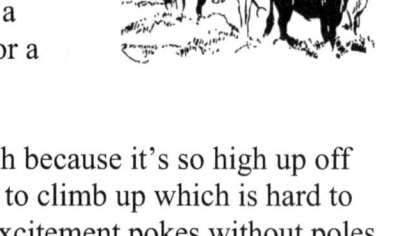

Accessing a good cow tail is difficult though because it's so high up off the ground that cowpokes need a poke pole to climb up which is hard to carry around. Many times for extra added excitement pokes without poles will wait for the cows to go to sleep, tip them, poke them, and get an exciting ride. If you last for more then eight seconds you are a winner.

Odd Fact:
Some cowpokes like to eat their cow tails shaved, and some like to eat them with the hair still on them. This appears to be a lifestyle choice.

Ingredients:
2-3 lbs. cow tails
2 bay leaves
Worcestershire sauce or soy sauce
Kosher salt
Fresh-cracked black pepper

Instructions:
Heat oven to 350 degrees.

Put cow tails in a shallow baking dish. Shake over several large splashes of Worcestershire or soy sauce. Sprinkle liberally with kosher salt and fresh-ground black pepper. Scatter the bay leaves on top and pour in water to come up to a scant 1/4 way up the meat. Cover the dish tightly with foil—tent it slightly, so the foil is not touching the meat.

Bake in the oven for at least two hours and check the meat. Fork 'n tender is not done enough for cow tail. Press the meat with your finger—if it's bouncy, it's not done.

After three hours, the meat should be darkly bronzed and yielding, even sticky to the touch just the way mom loves it. This is a good sign that the collagen has melted. (Very large cow tail pieces may take up to four hours, but I would encourage you to remove the little pieces after three hours.)

You could pull the meat and serve it on top of polenta, mashed potatoes, or creamy parmesan risotto. A bright and peppery green salad on the side would be nice.

Or you could just eat a bowl of them like a greedy peasant, huddled in a dark corner of the basement, sucking the meat off the bones as my husband does, and then moaning "Give me more!"

That's usually my choice.

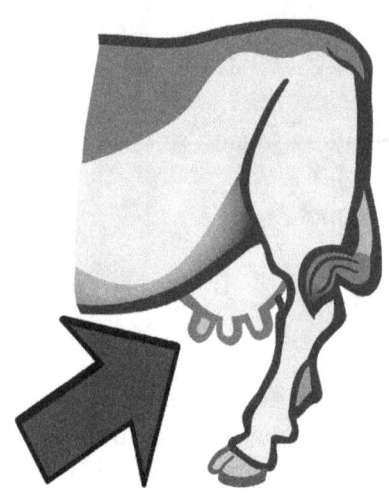

Udder Butter Cream
Cheesy Does It
Slickpoo, ID.

My husband thinks my snuggle puppies are the best! You probably think your double lattes are the best. Ok, so maybe he is biased, or he just hasn't tried your Congo bongos like everyone else in the city has… yet.

Last year, Rusty sure did a number on my teats. At one point they literally looked shredded. That's when I knew I had to get serious and do something more than a standard teat dip. That is when I found *Cheesy Does It* and their homemade Udder Butter Cream!

We're whipping up a batch right now as a natural body lotion for me and our sweet Jersey cows after milking time.

Ingredients:
¾ cup Coconut Oil
¾ cup Shea Butter
3 Tablespoons Sweet Almond Oil
1 ½ teaspoons Lanolin
2-4 Tablespoons Grated Beeswax (optional)
2 Tablespoons Arrowroot Powder

½ teaspoon Vitamin E
1 teaspoon Rosemary Infused Olive Oil
30 drops Lavender Essential Oil
30 drops Tea Tree Essential Oil

Instructions:
In a double boiler, melt the coconut oil, shea butter, lanolin, and beeswax.

Once it's combined, shut off the stove and let it sit, melted, for about half an hour and whisk in the arrowroot powder.

Set the bowl in another bowl of ice water to hasten the cooling process stirring occasionally, scraping the sides as it begins to harden.

Once about 2/3 of it is solid, use the whisk attachment of your mixer on high to whip it up until you get the right "whipped" texture. Add in the rosemary, lavender, and tea tree oil along with the Vitamin E and whisk it again.

Spoon into a container and, if possible, store between 50-80 degrees.

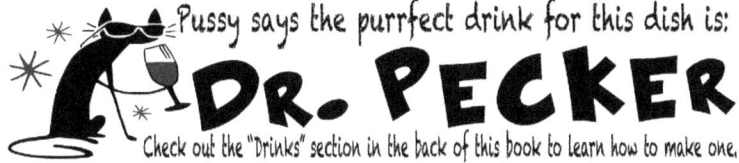

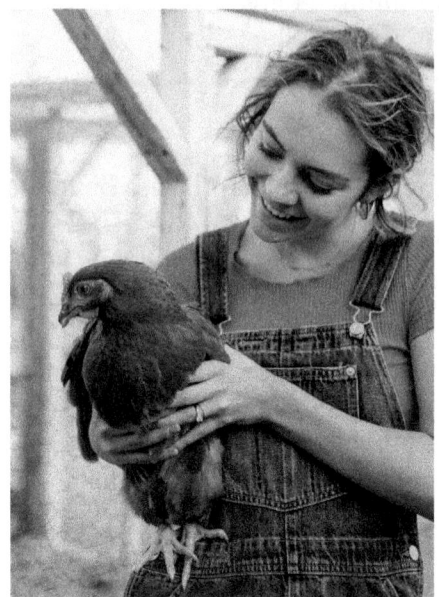

Chicken

A female chicken will mate with many different males. But if she decides after the deed is done that she doesn't want a particular rooster's offspring, she can eject his sperm. This is very similar to the human version of "spitting it out."

A chicken has not had the chance to work its muscles for very long, and so, the meat is very tender, it is not anywhere near as hard as a rooster. They also need much less beating and pounding than a hard cock to make them soft and tender.

While being a softer meat then a rooster, chickens are still preferred to be shot out of a gun to test airplane windows.

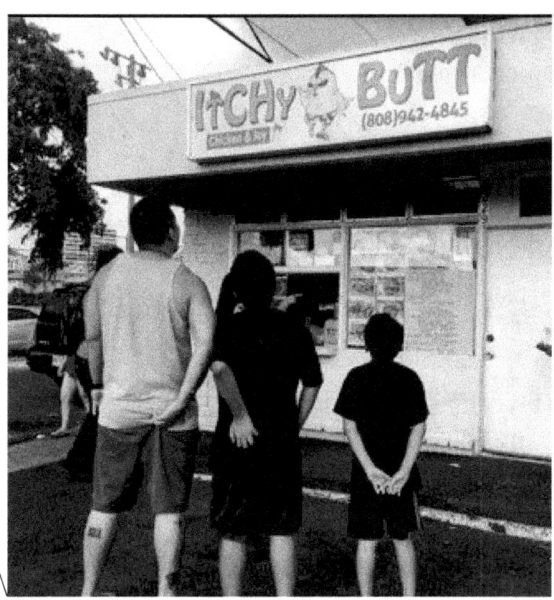

Dirty Rice – Dirty Chicken
Itchy Butt Chicken and Joy
Tightwad, MO.

Itchy butts...we all get them sometimes. But most of my itching comes from the dirty rice and not the chicken.

Some like their chicken really clean, but I like mine really dirty. So dirty I usually can't wait to get home because usually it doesn't smell all that great and it itches really bad. Believe me; I know why they call it *Itchy Butt*.

Pro Tip:
Don't ever ask your friends to share your Itchy Butt, nor should you share your friends when they ask. That's just not right!

Ingredients:
2 Tbs. vegetable oil
1 lb. chicken livers, finely minced (I use a mini food processor)
½ lb. ground pork or pork sausage crumbled
¾ cup minced green bell pepper (or substitute jalapeños for a spicier dish)
1 cup minced onion
¼ cup diced celery

1 Tbs. minced garlic
1 Tbs. Creole spice seasoning
1 tsp. Salt
1 tsp. Freshly ground black pepper
2 cups chicken or beef stock
3 bay leaves
5-6 cups cooked white rice
¼ cup minced fresh parsley

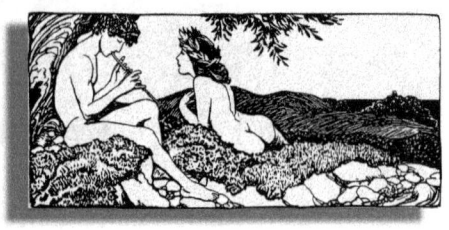

Instructions:
Crank up your favorite music. This is an essential step if you want to make authentic Itchy Butt dirty chicken. We all know where there's Itchy Butt there's going to be some squirming going on! You might as well look like your dancing, right?

In a large, deep skillet heat the vegetable oil over medium-high heat. Add the chicken livers and pork and cook, frequently stirring, until the meats are browned, 5-6 minutes.

Add the onions, green peppers, celery, garlic, Creole seasoning, salt, black pepper, and bay leaves and cook for about 5 minutes, stirring frequently.

Pour the stock into the pan and give it another good stir. Bring to a boil and simmer for 5 minutes or so.

Add the rice to the mixture and stir again. Continue to cook until the rice is heated through, about another 5 minutes.

Remove the bay leaves, stir in the diced parsley and serve it. You now have Itchy Butt! Tell your friends.

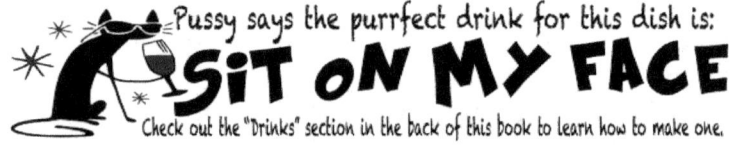

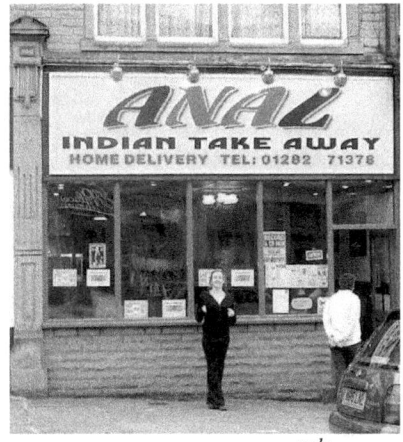
yelp

Aunt Fred's Breaded Chicken Arms
Anal Indian Takeaway
Tulsa, Ok.

Aunt Fred and his *Anal Indian Takeaway* is a real oddity in Tulsa.

Not a top-shelf drag queen name for sure. What is odd about Aunt Fred is his chicken motif fetish. He will wear a chicken feather boa, with a beak. He is always on the lookout for a few big, cock crazy guys that really want to drench him in their white gravy and eat him. Not that this is that weird of a thing for Tulsa.

What is weird is that Aunt Fred's mom is very understanding about all of this. What she really hates about her son Aunt Fred is the fact that he is also dyslexic. It is bad enough that he repetitively says racecar backwards, which is of course racecar. But what really angers his mom is when he accidently says Tulsa backwards and tells everyone he is from Aslut.

Ingredients:
2 lbs. Wings
1 cup Flour
1 heaping cup Panko bread crumb

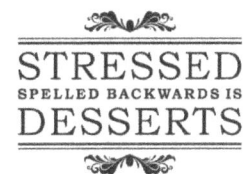

Season to taste with:
Cayenne Pepper
Black Pepper
Garlic Powder
2 Eggs

Sauce:
Crystal Buffalo Sauce
2 tbsp. Butter
Optional for Garlic Fiends: 3 cloves Garlic pressed or finely chopped

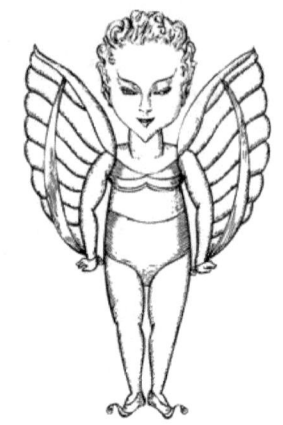

Instructions:
Preheat oven to 435°

Mix flour, panko bread crumbs, cayenne pepper, black pepper, and garlic powder in a bowl. Wisk the eggs in a separate bowl.

Cut up your cock. If using full wings just cut right through the joint, and you're done.

Dip your wings into eggs, then into the flour mixture. Pack the flour onto the wings for an extra crispy coating. Then put onto a well-greased pan. Cook your cock in the oven for 20 min. at 435°. Then turn over your wings and cook an additional 20 min. at 445°.

While that is cooking, you can prepare the sauce. Combine the buffalo sauce, butter, and garlic in a saucepan and warm on the stove.

Put sauce in a large preferably stainless steel bowl, add your wings and toss to coat them.

My mom made two dishes: Take it or Leave it.
  *- **Stephen Wright***

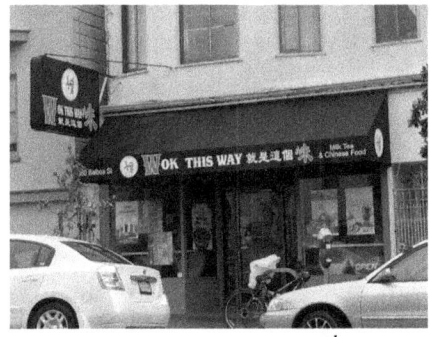
yelp

Lime Chicken & Sticky Honey Sauce
Wok This Way!
Boston, MA.

It's always the *"Same Old Song and Dance"* at the *"Wok This Way"* in Boston and *"I Don't Want to Miss a Thing"* when *"Out Go the Lights"*.

You can *"Make Love in an Elevator"* and get *"Back in the Saddle again"*. Be careful if the *"Dude Looks Like a Lady"*, because *"Janie's Got a Gun"* and you could be *"Livin on the Edge"*.

"Kiss Your Past Goodbye" when *"Lightning Strikes"* and you "*Get an Attitude Adjustment"*.

Do you know *"What Kind of Love Are You On"* when *"Kings and Queens"* *"Come Together"* , are *"Falling in Love"* and they *"Chip Away the Stone"*.

"What it takes" is for you to *"Shut up and dance"* and *"Let the Music do the Talking"* when you feel *"F.I.N.E"* and will *"Love Me Two Times"*.

The *"Crazy"* *"Blind Man"* with *"Nine Lives"* has such a *"Sweet Emotion"* when the *"Deuces are Wild"* and he gets the *"Rocking Phenomena"* and the *"Boogie Boogie Woogie Flu"*.

Ingredients:
1½ pounds boneless skinless chicken thighs (or breasts)
2 Tablespoons olive oil
1 teaspoon ground cumin
1 teaspoon chili powder
½ teaspoon salt
¼ teaspoon pepper
½ cup honey
Juice of one lime
Zest of one lime
2 Tablespoons soy sauce
1 garlic clove, minced

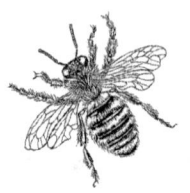

Instructions:
In a medium-sized skillet over medium heat add olive oil. In a small bowl combine cumin, chili powder, salt, and pepper. Rub on chicken and place in skillet. Cook for 3-4 minutes on each side or until chicken is no longer pink and 165 degrees. Remove chicken and set aside on a plate.

Add honey, lime juice, and zest (not the soap), soy sauce, and garlic. Bring to a boil over medium-high heat and reduce heat and whisk until it starts to thicken; about 2 minutes. Add the chicken back to the skillet and coat in the sauce. Garnish with lime wedges if desired.

Hometown Aerosmith fans are different from other Aerosmith fans, and that mainly has to do with Joe Perry. It's tough to overstate his strange grip on the local psyche. Tyler is a star who belongs to the whole world, but Perry, that dude belongs to Boston.

-Rob Sheffield

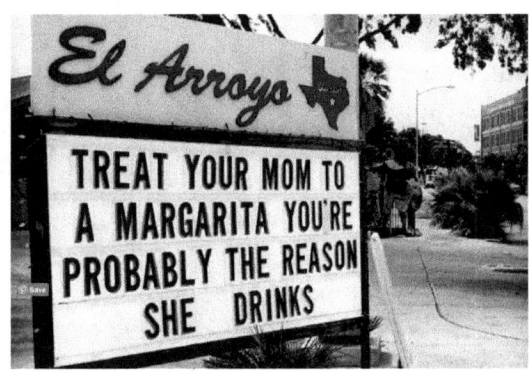
wideopencountry

Sticky Honey Breasts
El Arroyo
Spread Eagle, WI.

It's not just a great name for a "professional" dancer, it's a recipe!

I'd never had Sticky Honey Breasts before but now I'm hooked! I do two breasts up a week with all that goo… four on the weekends if my best friend Tabitha comes by. It's great because she's a big meat eater!

My mother always had Sticky Honey Breasts. Some say that's why dad married her. Well other then the fact nobody else wanted anything to do with him.

Ingredients:
2 pounds of chicken thighs wings (or breasts)
1 tablespoon olive oil
2 teaspoons sesame oil
1 teaspoon coarse salt

For the Sticky Honey Sauce you'll need
1/3 cup honey
2 tablespoons soy sauce
1 teaspoon sesame oil
1 tablespoon grated fresh ginger
2 cloves garlic minced
1 lime juiced

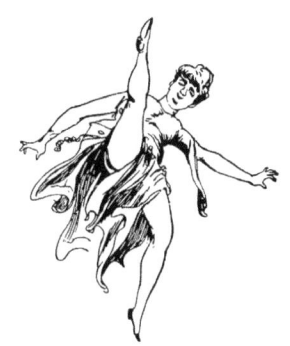

2 Sliced green onions for garnish
2 teaspoons Sesame seeds for garnish
Serve with rice and steamed broccoli

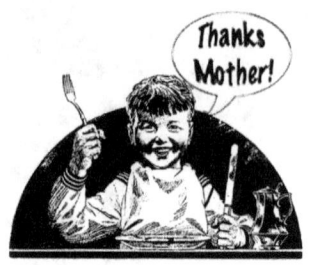

Instructions:
Preheat oven to 400 degrees.

Line a baking sheet with parchment paper or foil for easy cleanup. Wash and pat dry chicken. Toss with 1 tablespoon olive oil and 2 teaspoons sesame oil. Arrange on a prepared baking sheet and sprinkle with coarse salt.

Bake for 20-25 minutes or until internal temperature reaches 165 degrees.

While chicken is baking, quit jacking around and make your sauce!

For Sticky Sauce:
Add all ingredients to the medium-size saucepan. (you want something a bit bigger so your sauce will reduce quicker).

Bring to a simmer and cook. Occasionally stirring, until reduced by half and you are left with about 1/3 of a cup of sauce. Approximately 10 minutes or so.

Toss cooked chicken in with the sauce. Garnish with sesame seeds and sliced green onion, serve with rice and let your Sticky Honey Breast party begin!

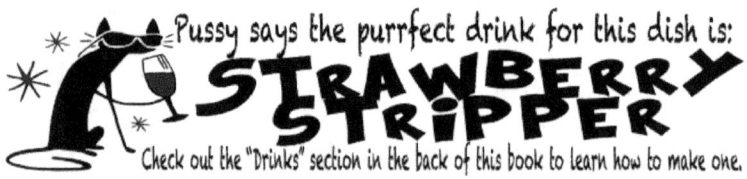

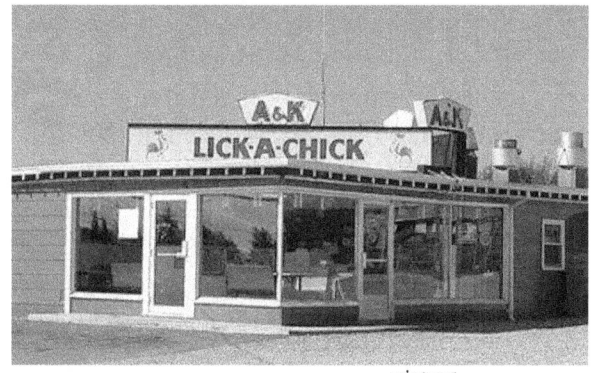
pintrest

Chicken Breasts & Creamy BBC
Lick A Chick Restaurant
Eel Pie Island, River Thames

I've traveled all over the world and always wanted to lick up the world-famous Chicken Breasts & Creamy BBC Sauce at the *Lick-A-Chick*.

Lick-A-Chick is located on the River Thames and is not only noted for its chicken pot breasts but also for its BBC (Black Bean & Cream) sauce.

This thick white cream cheese sauce dripping down the heaving breasts with BBC in between them is an unforgettable sight. It is so good you may never want to put the breasts in your mouth again.

Ingredients:
4 -5 boneless chicken breasts
1 can black beans
1 package cream cheese
1 can corn
1 jar missing finger salsa

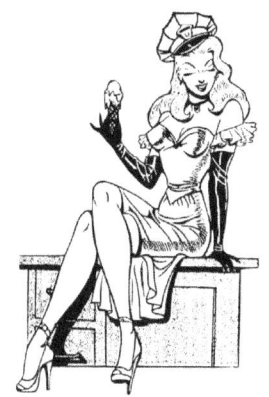

Instructions:
Take 4-5 frozen, boneless chicken breasts put into a crock pot. Add 1 can of black beans, drained, 1 jar of salsa and 1 can of corn drained.

Keep in crock pot on high for about 4-5 hours or until chicken is cooked.

Add 1 package of cream cheese (just throw it on top!) and let sit for about 1/2 hour. Eat up!

My doctor told me to stop having intimate dinners for four unless there are three other people.
   - **Orson Welles**

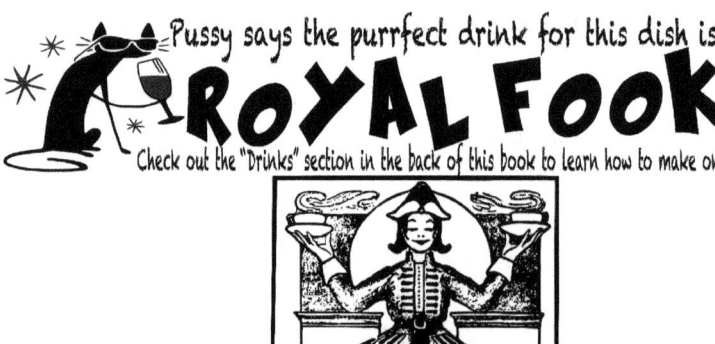

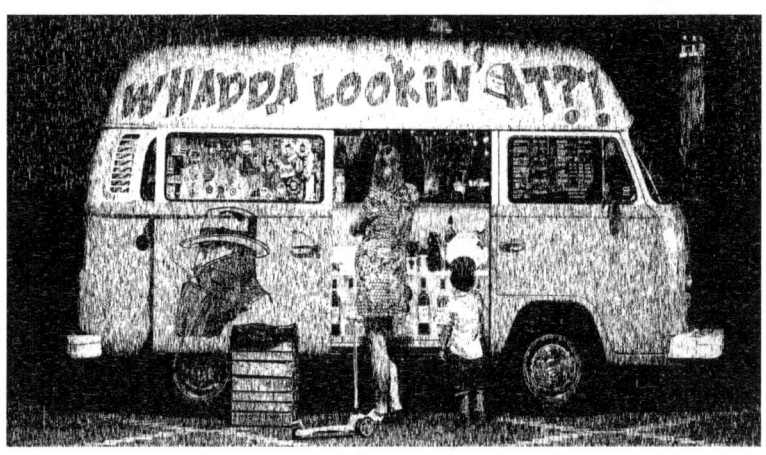

Big Breasts -N- Taquitos
Whadda Lookin' At?! Food Truck
New York, NY (Down by da Docks)

Even though I am a female, I just love "Big Breasts!" Big Breasts are enjoyed by both men and women of all ages and Sweaty Betty has enough for everyone.

Now as all boys learn in Junior High, the correct way to calculate a breasts volume for a hemispherical bra cup is:

$$V = \frac{2\pi r^3}{3} \qquad V = \frac{\pi D^3}{12}$$

And if the cup is a hemi-ellipsoid, its volume is given by the formula:

$$V = \frac{2\pi abc}{3} \qquad V \approx \frac{\pi \times cw \times cd \times wl}{12}$$

Cups, of course, give a hemispherical shape to breasts and underwires give shape to cups. So the curvature radius of the underwire is the key parameter to determine the volume and weight of the breast.

To help out, I have included the following chart from the fine folks at bigbustsupport.com:

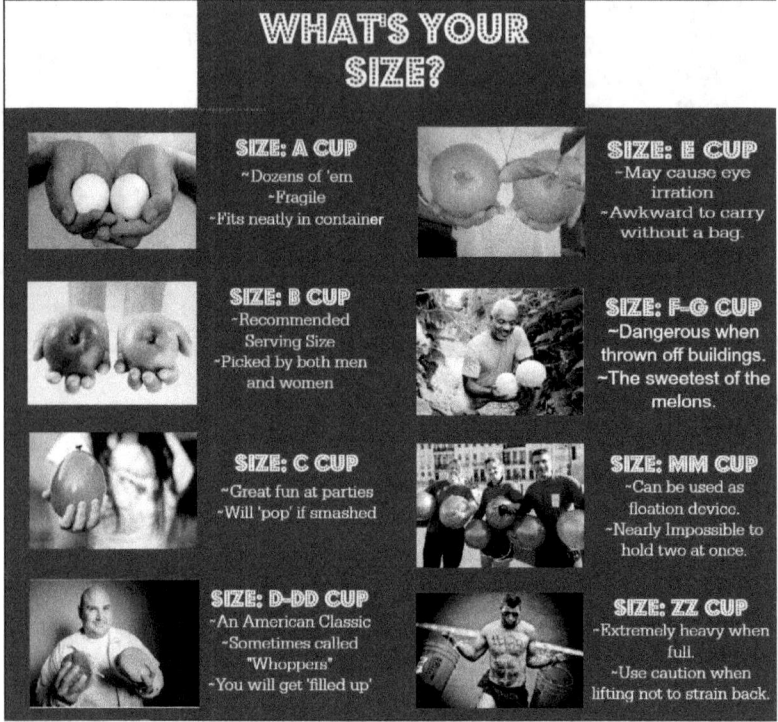

Taking all of this into account and to make a long story short, Sweaty Betty is a whopping zz cup.

Now when she was in the Navy, they called her Naval Nipples. Not because of her service, but because of where on her body her nipples hung down to. Yes her breasts resemble a tube sock with an orange in it, but the guys all still dig 'em.

Anyhow Sweaty Betty's food truck got its name from Betty always yelling at her customer's *"Whadda You Looking At"?*

Ingredients:
10 oz. Canned 98% fat-free chunk white chicken breast in water.
1/2 cup salsa

1/3 cup shredded fat-free cheddar cheese
1/4 tsp. taco seasoning mix
Eight 6-inch corn tortillas
Optional dips: red enchilada sauce, additional salsa, fat-free sour cream.

Instructions:
Preheat oven to 375 degrees. Spray a baking sheet with nonstick spray.

In a medium bowl, mix chicken with salsa. Cover and refrigerate for 15 minutes.

Drain any excess liquid from the chilled chicken mixture. Stir in cheese and taco seasoning. Place tortillas between 2 damp paper towels. Microwave for 1 minute, or until warm and pliable.

One at a time spread each tortilla with 1/8th of chicken mixture, about 2 tbsp.; tightly roll up into a tube, place on the baking sheet, seam side down, and secure with toothpicks if needed.

Bake until crispy, 14 to 16 minutes. (Don't worry if they crack and "explode" a little!) Eat up! Makes 4 servings.

"I love Thanksgiving turkey...it's the only time in Los Angeles that you see natural breasts."
   - Arnold Schwarzenegger

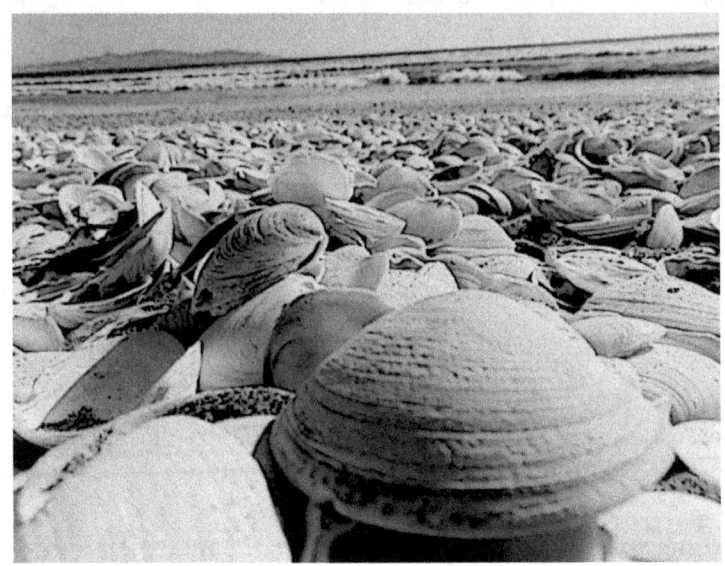

Clams & Oysters

When people think of clams, they probably think of a nice hot bowl of clam chowder or other seafood dishes. What you never think about is how old they are.

Some clams are among the longest-lived species in the world. For example, in 2007, scientists discovered a specimen of the ocean quahog that was between 405 and 410 years old. Giant Clams live about 150 years while Cold Seep Clams don't even reach maturity until they are 100.

Now think about that the next time you worry about how old your clams are.

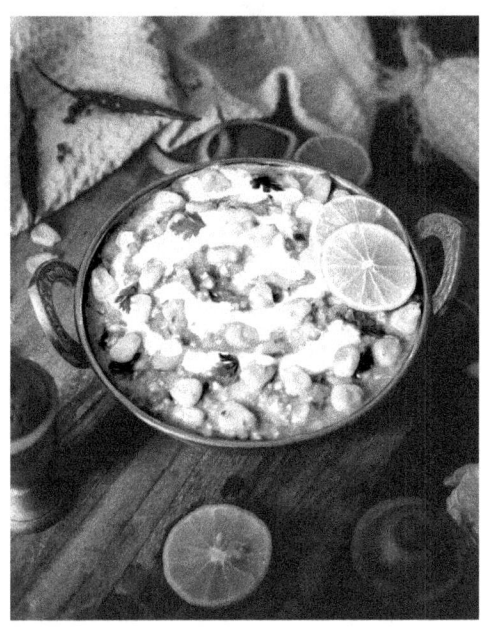

Hot Noodle Deep in White Clam Sauce
The Munch Box
Virgin, Utah

Virgin Utah is not necessarily a place that you would expect to find the best clams and oysters drenched in a fine white sauce. But at the *Munch Box,* you can find many older bearded clams all nice and ready to be sauced up.

I used canned baby clams in addition to fresh littlenecks in this pasta, but you could easily use one or the other. If you want to omit the canned clams, stir about a half cup of fish stock into the sauce.

You'll also want to be sure to slice the garlic, not mince it. This will allow it to melt into the sauce and will give you a sweet, mellow flavor rather than a bitter one.

Ingredients:
8 ounces dry linguini
2 tbs. olive oil
1/2 small onion, minced
1 head garlic, sliced
A pinch dried hot red pepper flakes
A pinch dried oregano
8 tbs. dry white wine
1/2 can baby clams, plus juice
12 littleneck clams, scrubbed well
1 tbs. butter, cut into small pieces
1/3 cup chopped fresh parsley
salt and pepper to taste

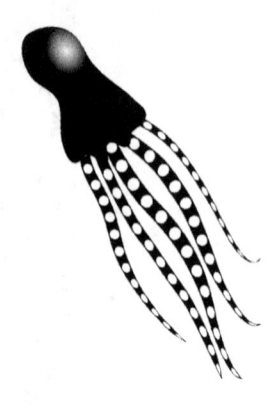

I used fresh littlenecks in addition to canned baby clams in this pasta, but you could easily use one or the other. If you want to omit the canned clams, stir about a half cup of fish stock into the sauce.

You'll also want to be sure to slice the garlic, not mince it. This will allow it to melt into the sauce and will give you a nice, mellow flavor rather than a bitter one.

Instructions:
Prepare the linguini noodles according to the directions of the package.

While that cooks, heat the oil in a large skillet or pot set over medium-high heat. Add the onion and sauté until it begins to soften. Add the garlic, red pepper, and oregano and cook for 1 minute, taking care not to burn the garlic.

Stir in the wine (the sauce will turn white as you add it!) and the liquid from the baby clams. Cook for a few minutes to allow the flavors to come together.

Add the littlenecks, cover, and steam for about 5 minutes or until the clams open. Stir in the baby clams and cook until just heated through. Remove from heat and set aside the littlenecks. Stir in the butter and parsley. Season to taste with salt and pepper.

Drain the pasta and return it to the pot.

Add the sauce to the pasta and toss to coat. Top with little necks.

Then play with the hot wet clams with your fingers, your lips and tongue. I promise you'll have no complaints about doing a lot of that from anyone.

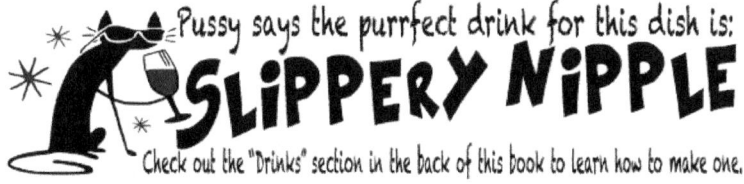

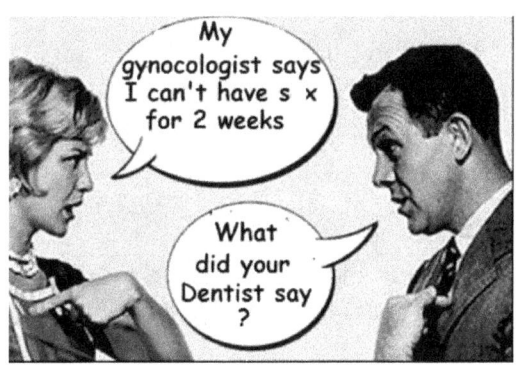

Crazyhyena

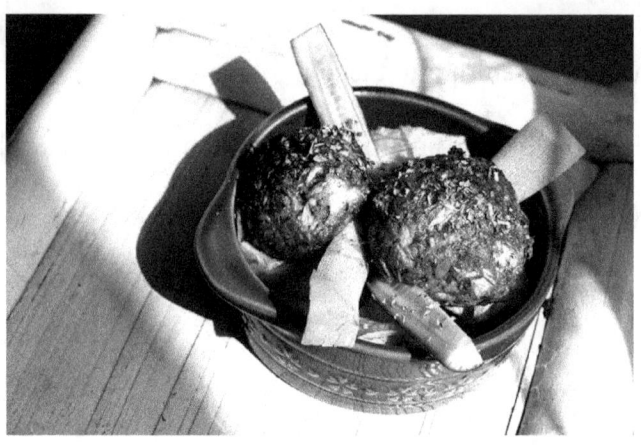

RMO (Rocky Mountain Oysters)
Stoner's Paradise
Loveland, Colorado

Smoking 420, eating Rocky Mountain Oysters, downing a few beers with a few sisters is a college girl's right to passage in the Rockies. At *Stoner's Paradise* in Loveland Colorado introducing young ladies into eating big browned bull balls has become a tradition.

If you make this recipe be sure to ask your butcher for calf testicles NOT bull testicles! Calf testicles are the size of a walnut and are much more tender than the larger bull testicles. But if you prefer larger and tougher balls go for the bull.

Use enough vegetable oil to fill your frying container halfway to the top to allow for bubbling up and splattering of oil on your testicles. Make sure to completely cover your testicles, clams or funbags while frying or cooking bacon naked for that matter.

Ingredients:
2 pounds calf testicles This should be a dozen or so. Question your butcher if he tries to sell you only two testicles. He may be giving you a bag of bull.
4 beers and a cup of Tequila (You'll need at least two beers and the Tequila to drink while yer cooking!)

2 eggs, beaten
1 1/2 cups all-purpose flour
1/4 cup yellow cornmeal
Salt and ground black pepper to taste
Vegetable oil
1 tablespoon hot pepper sauce

Instructions:
With a very sharp knife, split the tough skin sack that surrounds each of your testicles. Try not to have too many weird thoughts as you remove the skin (you can remove the skin easily if you freeze your balls in advance and peel the skin away as they thaw).

Either leave each ball whole or slice them into approximately 1/4- to 1/2-inch-thick ovals. Place slices in a large pan or blow with enough beer to cover them and let sit 2 hours.

In a shallow bowl, combine eggs, flour, cornmeal, salt, and pepper in preparation to smear on those balls like a pro. Remove your balls from the beer; drain and then press them firmly into the bowl filled with the coating mixture. Have fun Rolling 'em around some until they're completely covered.

In a large, deep pot heat oil to 375°. Deep fry your balls for 3 minutes or until golden brown. If your balls were golden brown or darker to start with just make them a color darker. Then drain your testicles and place them on paper towels.

Never fondle your testicles! Don't play with them or show 'em in public. Just poke them with a fork and put them in your mouth until your mouth is overcome by hot juices. And as the saying goes, "Wipe your chin and do it again!" Share them with your friends or anyone who'll dare to put them steamy hot RMOs in their mouths.

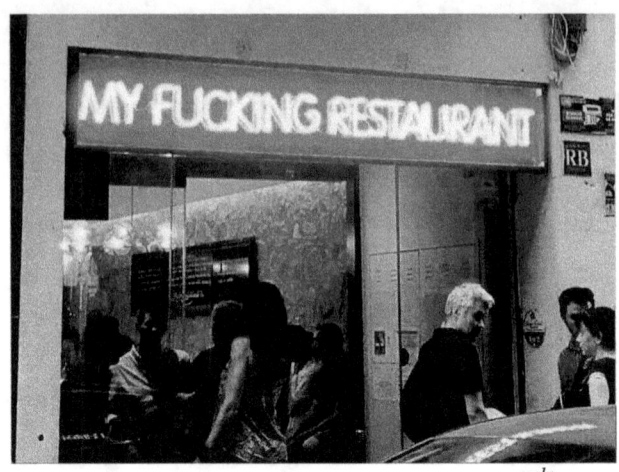
yelp

Drunken Clams & Sausage
My Fucking Restaurant
Cincinnati, Ohio

"Even though a friend of mine was murdered here while we were eating I really do recommend the Drunken Clams.
    –*Ibea Cummin,* Cincinati, Ohio

Ingredients:
2 tablespoons olive oil
1-pound spicy Italian sausage, removed from casing
2 shallots, minced
1 (medium-sized) head of fennel, sliced
2 cloves garlic, minced
1 cup dry white wine
1 cup low sodium chicken stock
2 dozen littleneck clams, rinsed and cleaned
1/2 cup heavy cream

Instructions:
In a large skillet set over medium heat add olive oil. Once the oil is hot mix in your sausage and begin to brown it if it isn't all ready. Break up the sausage as it cooks. Add in shallots and fennel.

Continue cooking until the vegetables start to soften, and your sausage is no longer pink. Add in the garlic and cook until fragrant, about 30 seconds. Now add in white wine and cook down halfway.

Pour in chicken stock and stir to combine. Place cleaned raw clams on top of the mixture, slightly pushing them into the stock. Cover and let cook for about 8 minutes or until completely opened. If any clams do not open, throw them away.

Carefully remove the opened clams from the dish and add white cream to the sausage mixture. Cook for 5 minutes and either add the clams back to the dish for serving or divide your clams equally between bowls and pour the hot sausage/broth mixture over the top.

* Want to learn how to clean your clams? Read all about it in my beer steamed clams recipe.
* Prep time includes the time it takes to clean as many of the clams you can eat.

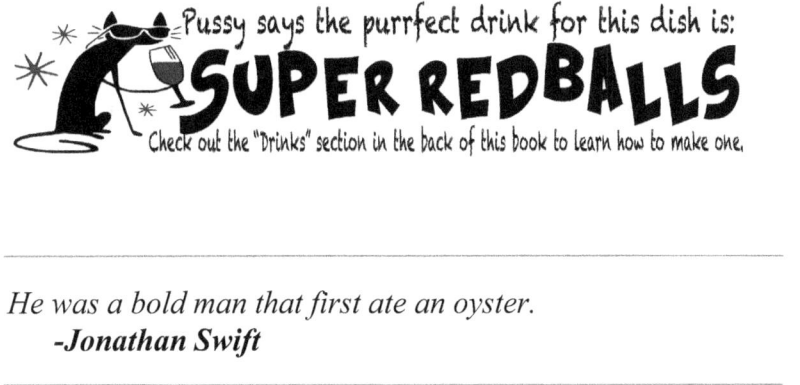

Pussy says the purrfect drink for this dish is: **SUPER REDBALLS**
Check out the "Drinks" section in the back of this book to learn how to make one.

He was a bold man that first ate an oyster.
   -Jonathan Swift

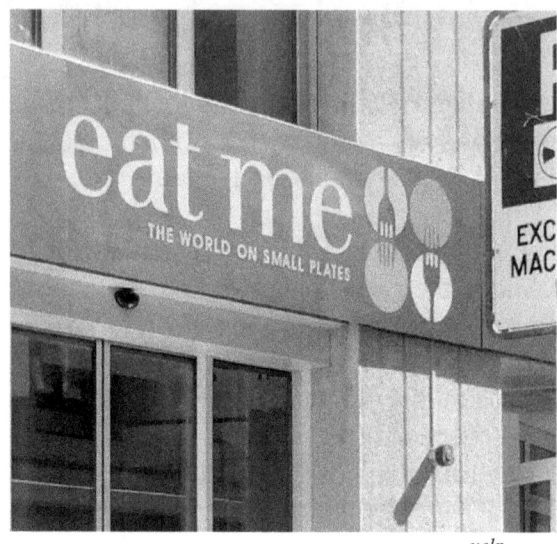
yelp

BEER STEAMED CLAMS
EAT ME
CINCINNATI, OHIO

There is nothing more enjoyable than eating out your favorite beer-soaked clam on a dinner table. Just thinking of the sight of a well cleaned naked, spread wide open clam sitting on the dinner table in front of you excites men and many women. Especially both before and after dinner.

I often invite my female friends over for a clam soak. It is much like a day at the spa.

If you have never soaked your clam in beer, don't worry, it tickles and feels really great. As you soak your clam, be sure to get rid of all the sand in it. Nothing is worse than biting into a clam and getting sand in your mouth. Gross.

After all of us girls get our clams' soaked we get them steaming hot by lovingly mixing a little garlic into some olive oil and smear it right onto our clams. We then rub them until those babies open wide up. We finish off our clams with generous streams of butter.
When we get around to devouring each other's clams we first dip soft bread in them to soak up the juice. Sweet baby Jesus it's incredible; all

those soaked clams on our dinner table excites both me, my husband and all our friends. What a wonderful clamfest.

Pro Tip:
If a clam won't open, don't eat it. How easy is that?

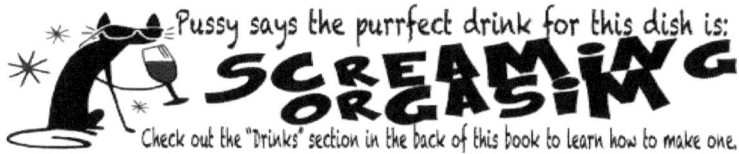

"The most remarkable thing about my mother is that for thirty years she served the family nothing but leftovers. The original meal has never been found."
  - ***Calvin Trillin***

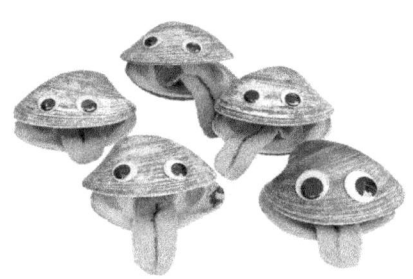

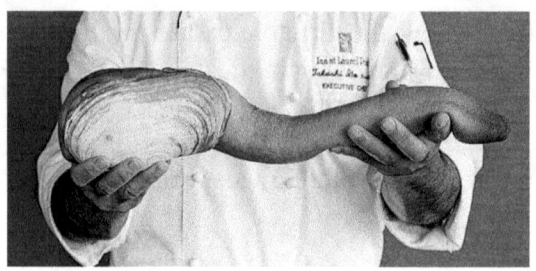
carolinewest

Long Dong Squirt & Tequila
Long Dong Silvers
Ballsalla
Isle Of Man

Geoducks are just weird. Like most things long and round there are so many things you can do with them. Some have tried to eat them. The usual reaction is "That's sofa king is not going into my mouth?!"

Fortunately at *Long Dong Silvers* someone was drunk enough on Tequila to try one. Between the saline injections and projectile vomiting in the ambulance it was a pity that he was not able to report what it tasted like.

Safety Tip: Your geoduck, should be completely dead when you buy it with no bad odor. DO NOT let someone slip you a live one! You should be careful in that even though it is dead, it still may try to attack you!

Ingredients:
1 Dead geoduck, cleaned and sliced thin
2 cloves garlic, minced
2 tablespoons fresh Lime Juice
3 tablespoons Olive Oil
6 ounces of Tequila
3 tablespoons Fresh Cilantro, chopped
1/4 teaspoon Ground Red Pepper
1 Yellow Pepper
4-6 Bamboo Skewers, soaked in water

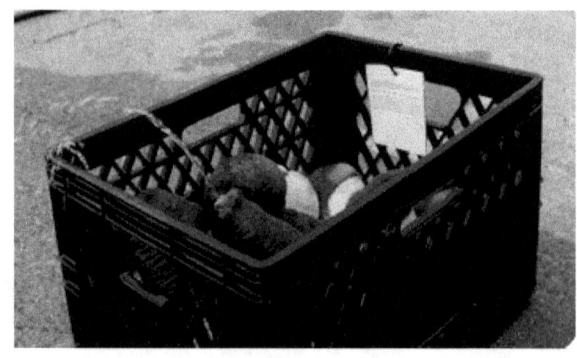

How to Clean a Geoduck:

Safety Tip! Be careful because the geoduck will squirt at you even after it is dead, so be sure to wear some safety glasses!

Cut the geoduck out of its shell. Use a sharp knife and be ready to kill it again. Be sure that you get all the tender meat off of the inside. Remove the shell and all of its guts.

See that big round thing? That is its stomach. If you are adventurous, you can cut it open and eat something out of it that this thing ate days ago and it has not killed or digested yet. Like those skinny, little, translucent worm-like things or all those miniature, moving crabs about the size of fleas.

If you wish you can add all those live little things to chowder or soup. If you have not been successful in killing them they will reproduce in the warm, wet chowder or in your stomach so be prepared for something to crawl out of your bowl.

Now pour scolding hot water over the geoduck entrails, focusing on the areas covered in skin. If anything is still moving, kill it with even more scolding hot water. The skin should easily peel off just like a prom dress.

Once you get the skin off, pour more scolding hot water on it to make sure you really have actually killed it.

Safety Tip! A great way to check if it is still alive is to submerge the now excoriated geoduck under scolding hot water to see if it jumps or moves. If so hold it there until it stops moving and you once again kill it.

Everything that has now not crawled off of the plate or out of the pan, and remains laying still is now probably edible.

How to Cook a Geoduck:
After drinking a shot of the tequila, dice the peppers into 1-inch pieces Toss the geoduck, garlic, lime juice, olive oil, cilantro, red pepper, and salt in a bowl. Refrigerate for 30 minutes while checking for movement.

Preheat an outdoor grill for high heat and lightly oil grate. Drain the water from the geoduck and discard. Never drink geoduck juice or water plants with it. Spear the geoduck pieces and pepper on the skewers.

Safety Tip! If one of the pieces flinches when stabbed throw it down the garbage disposal and turn it on as fast as you can. Pour 1% scalding water mixed with 99% sulfuric acid down the drain immediately. We are totally green here and don't want these things living in our nations sewer systems.

Cook on the searing hot grill until the geoduck turns opaque, about 5-6 minutes.

Mix up a very strong margarita with the remaining tequila, there is no other way to get this crap down your throat!

Safety Tip! If you feel something trying to crawl back up your throat, don't play with it! Either throw it up into a running garbage disposal or chug it down some scolding water immediately.

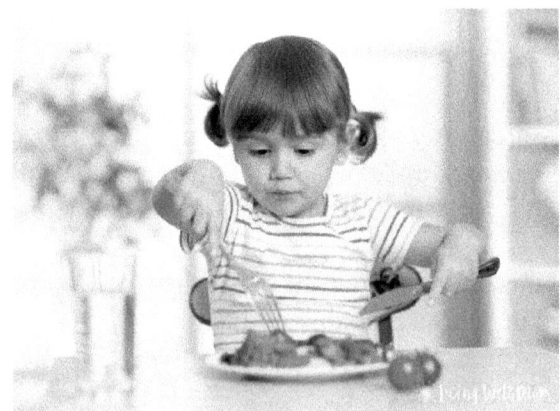

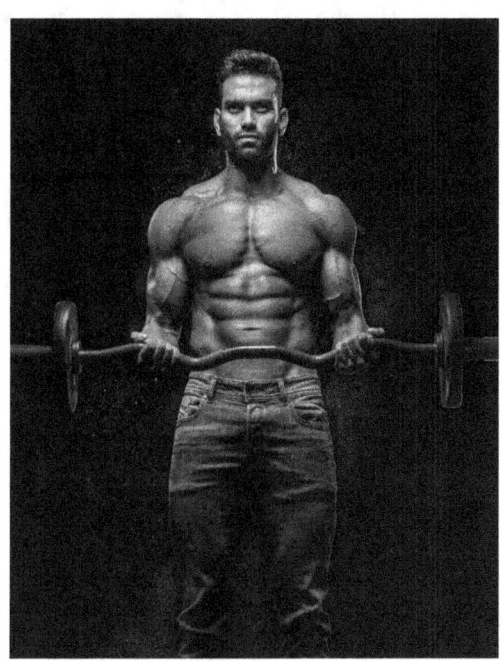

WIENERS, TUBE STEAKS & OTHER LOW HANGING MEATS

After the steaks, chops, breasts, ribs, thighs, hams, tenderloins and briskets are removed, there's a fair amount of gristle, fat, and offal remaining on a butchered animal. Early on, people realized this could be put to good use. One of these uses other than dog food is the American hot dog.

Hot dogs contain about 50 percent water and only 10 percent meat. That meat often consists of skeletal muscle such as bone, collagen, blood vessels, entrails, assholes, lips and cartilage.

Bon Appetite

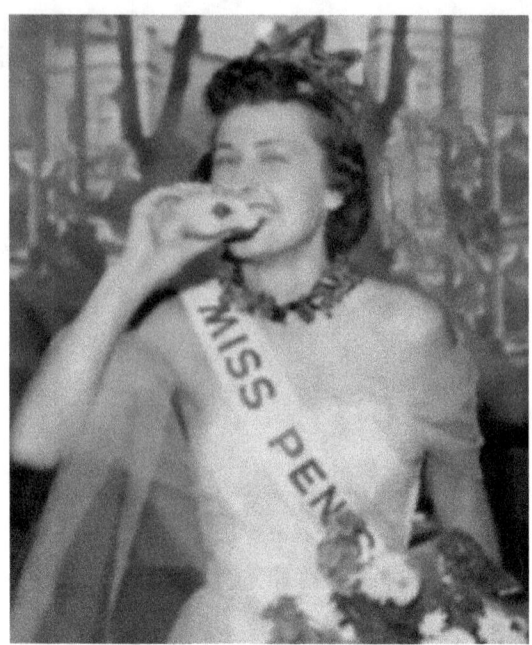

Sheboygan Press
Miss Pennsylvania enjoying a Sheboygan Slammer.

SHEBOYGAN SLAMMERS
THE SHEBOYGAN SLAMMER QUEEN
SHEBOYGAN, WI.

Most all of us have heard of the Johnsonville famous racing sausages at Miller Park. But have you heard of their less famous little sister *The Sheboygan Slammer Queen* and the festivities that go on around her?

I am here to tell you that every year the people of Sheboygan celebrate their world-famous tubes of meat by having the "Sheboygan Slammer Queen" Parade.

In fact, it is the highest honor for a girl to be crowned the "Sheboygan Slammer Queen." This lucky gal gets to ride around town sitting in a convertible with her top down so everyone can see her in her car.

After the parade, she would go back out to walk the streets and pick out the biggest, best and tastiest Slammers in town. Sometimes she would eat them with mustard and sometimes without anything on it. Occasionally she would ask the people to put their slammers into her bun.

By the end of the day the Slammer Queen would have looked at, felt, and tasted most all of the lovely meat tubes in town. This is a very time consuming, tiring endeavor. However, it is a very rewarding day for a young woman and causes a lot of jealousy amongst other women both married and single in town.

Fun fact:
Single mother of four Martha Rutherford won the coveted Sheboygan Slammer Queen Award five years in a row! Rumor has it she really impressed the judges by eating more tube steaks than any other woman in town.

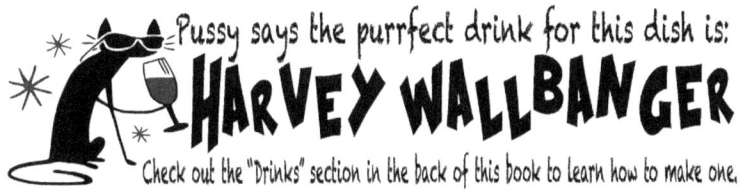

Hitting a golf ball correctly is the most sophisticated and complicated maneuver in all of sports, with the possible exception of eating a hot dog at a ball game without getting mustard on your shirt.
    -Ray Fitzgerald

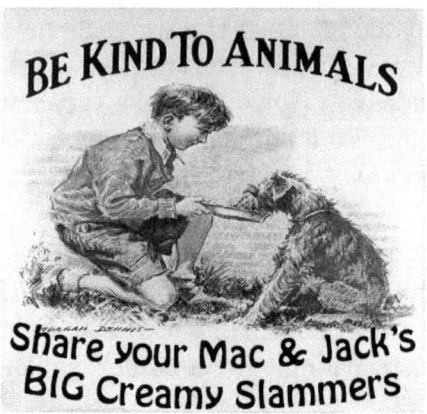

Mac's & Jack's BIG Creamy Slammers
Like No Udder
Milwaukee, Wisconsin

Wisconsin is famous for cutting the cheese. *Like No Udder* is renowned for their Mac' & Jack's Big Creamy Slammers.

Unlike most recipes in this book this one totally sucks. My dad use to make big batches of this crap and would freeze it. Before he went to work in the morning, he would put this shit in the oven on timed bake for us kids to eat after school. Sometimes it would be cold, and sometimes it would be burnt. It was never right.

We would always tell our hard working dad we loved it and ate it all, which was never the case and we would have to get rid of all the evidence. It was way too much for the garbage disposal to handle, so we use to feed it to the dog. The dog got tired of, the toilet would not handle it, so we would have to bury it in the back yard.

Sometimes dad would make Bennie Weenie with wine for us. The dog would always fall down the stairs. Not cool.

Ingredients:
1 1/2 cups macaroni
3/4 cup milk,
1 1/4 teaspoons dry mustard
1 1/4 teaspoons salt
1/8 teaspoon pepper
2 1/2 cups cheddar cheese
1 1/2 lbs. deli-Style frankfurters

Instructions:
Cook the macaroni in boiling salted water until tender. Drain and rinse in hot water.

Mix the milk, mustard, salt, pepper and 2 cups of the cheddar cheese into the top of a double boiler stirring frequently. Cook until the cheddar is melted and sauce is smooth. Mix in the macaroni.

Open face the slammers lengthwise and fill with the macaroni mixture. Sprinkle with more shredded cheddar and bake in a 400-degree oven for 15 minutes.

"This was gonna be great. WARNING! Never leave a full bowl of Mac'& Jacks Big Creamy Big Slammers sitting around any pet that can jump up on the table unless you want to pay for the pizza to get delivered.

-Danny's "In the doghouse" Donahue

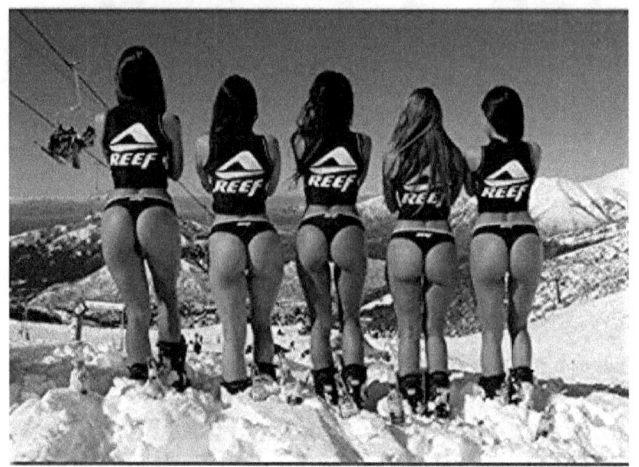
Sava Amazon.com

How's Your AssBeen?
(Smokin' Hot Round Bottoms)
Slope Side Meets
Aspen, Colorado

I have been sampling very many of the succulent *Smokin' Hot Round Bottoms* that are always on display at *Slope Side Meets* in Asbeen Colorado. People there openly display their round bottoms that they bring in with them from all over the world.

You can get any type of meat you like at Slope Side Meets; Cock, beaver, clams, creamed ham, wieners, hooters, and fried eggs.

With the large weekly rotating selection of new fresh bottoms, you never have to worry about eating the same round bottom twice.

Ingredients:
1 Round Bottom
1/4 TSP Garlic Powder
1/4 TSP Onion Powder
1 TSP Paprika
1/2 TSP Cayenne Pepper
Apple Chips

Instructions:
Rub your round bottom with olive oil and sit it into a bowl containing the homemade rub...50/50 Kosher Salt Pepper (4 TBS each Salt & Pepper)

Stick your bottom into the smoker at 225° and check your little apple chips every hour.

Smoke your meat for about three hours until done.

If you do not have a meat smoker at your house ask a friend to smoke your bottom for you!

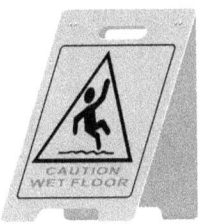

It's gonna get juicy in there so make sure you bring your

Rubbers!

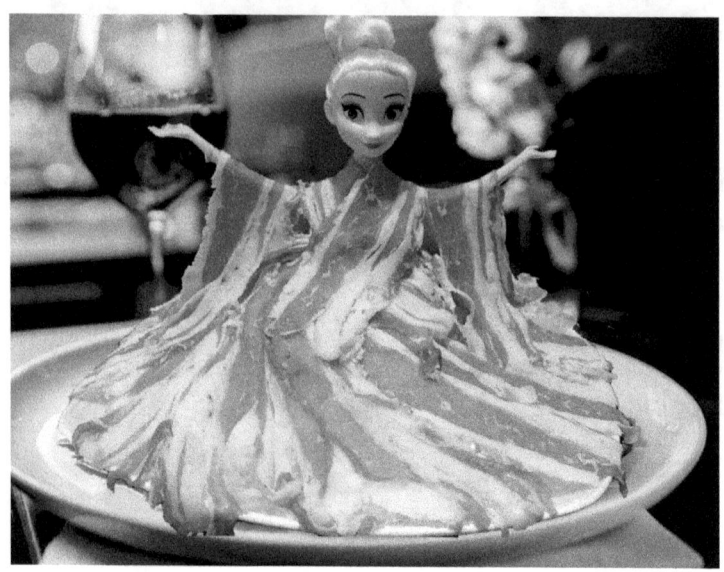

Korean BBQ Meat Doll
Just Falafs
Keister, West Virginia

One of my favorite types of restaurant niches in the world is Korean barbecue. Especially when the barbecue is built into the table itself.

There is something about being able to cook your own meat to your own exact doneness quickly at your table that makes for an excellent dining experience. The meat is so tasty coming right off the grill.

I was sitting on my keister in *Just Falafs* enjoying some fresh Korean cock on a bamboo skewer when they presented me with this unusual way to display their pork belly strips.

Yes she is wearing something underneath.

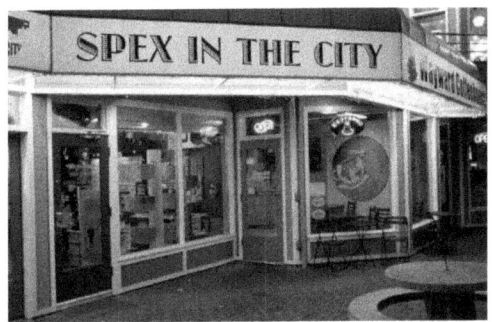
yelp

Perfect Prime Rib
Spex In The City
Florida Keys. FL.

A local legend, this place is smack dab in the middle of town and has more big meat swinging around in there than the next five butcher shops combined.

They have it all! Just run down the entire food-chain and they probably got a big, fat, smoked slab of it in there somewhere; hunky ribs so thick they'll put a dent in your couch and make your whole body shake for up to forty-eight hours! But they're most famous for the Big Meats Prime Rib.

FUN FACT:
It's called "prime rib" until you slide it in an oven, then it's a "roast." because you've roasted it. That same slab of meat can be ground up, in which case it is then called "hamburger." Tell your friends. It's golden tidbits like this that'll make you the real life of any party.

Ingredients:
1 prime rib; 3 bone minimum but no bigger than four bones unless you are cooking in a smoker.
3 oz of Kosher Salt, as needed
3 oz of Black pepper, ground
3 oz of dried garlic powder
4 sprigs Rosemary, as needed
Garlic, crushed, about 4 to six cloves as needed
2.2 oz Herbs, fresh, such as rosemary and thyme
1.1 oz whole Black peppercorns

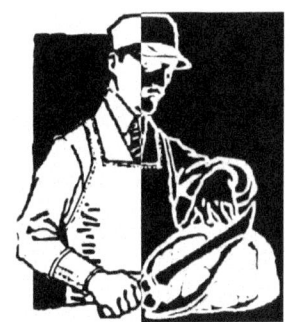

1 oz of dry mustard powder
2 - 4 Egg white
1 l Beef Stock
2 oz of prime rib rub or other type of dry rub (optional)

Instructions:
Preparation of your meat prior to cooking:

Unwrap your prime rib but keep the butcher paper to use as a cutting board for later on.

Mix your rub mixture in a separate dish and then rub your seasoning all over your meat. Slowly then faster and faster! Place roast in either a 2 gallon zip lock or oven roasting bag. Seal your roast in preparation for cooking

Place Prime Rib in a dish and let it sit for a minimum of 2 hours to up to as long as 12 hours. Great time to grab a nap, play with the dog or walk the kids.

Set up the immersion circulator or sous vide oven to accommodate the size of your meat. To determine how much water, place the roast in water to determine the water level.

To figure out the cook time, multiply the number of pounds by a multiplier of 2 to 2.5 hours then check the sundial and let the cat out. When water temperature reaches 80% readiness, go ahead and place your roast in the water bath.

Cook your roast to the (Ding!) You can leave it in the bath up to about an hour before texture changes towards a higher temperature.

Finishing:
About 30 - 45 minutes before the roast is finished, preheat your oven to 425 degrees.

In a small mixing bowl, crack two eggs and separate the yolk from the egg white. **NOTE:** you can also use pre-made egg whites if needed.

Take two sprigs of rosemary and chop them up finely. In a separate bowl combine the peppercorns, garlic powder and rosemary.

When the roast is finished, remove it from the bath and place the roast on a baking sheet that will be used for searing in the oven. Pat the roast dry to remove any moisture from cooking

Pour the remaining juices into a container to be used to make the au jus.

In a skillet, with a pat of butter, add minced garlic, black pepper, cooking liquid and ⅓ cup of beef broth. Bring to a boil and then simmer till the liquid is reduced by half. Skim off any solids and then pour reduction into a serving dish.

With a rubber spatula, cover the roast with egg white mixture. This is the binder to hold the dry ingredients for the crust.

Salt the prime rib and then liberally coat it with the dry mixture and cover as much as possible on the top, ends and sides.

Place prime rib in the pre-heated oven for 10-20 minutes until crust is a golden brown. Watch this process as to not "scorch" the crust.

Remove the roast after the allotted time and let "rest" for 15 minutes.

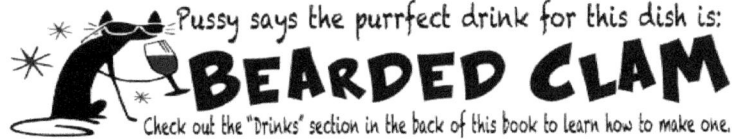

Pussy says the purrfect drink for this dish is: **BEARDED CLAM**
Check out the "Drinks" section in the back of this book to learn how to make one.

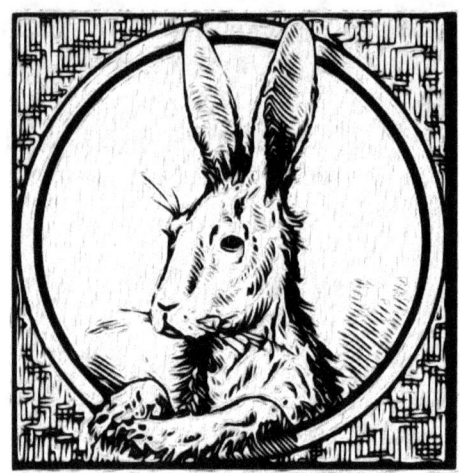

"Only serve one rabbit! Never one hare. Finding one hare in one's food, really pisses off one."
                    -**Recent Indian Proverb**

Roger Rabbit Ragu
Lettuce Eat
Bangalore, India

It's hot, it's traffic-jammed, it's air filled with the smells of local food shops on top of food shops on top of other food shops on top of house, huts and what seems to be a billion motor scooters, bikes, and carts.

Bangalore has 12 million people, and it seemed like they've all decided there the same day as me! It could take a week to get in! So we wait. I can't say I blame them a bit. The rabbit is to die for!

Ingredients:
1 big bunny
4 eggs
Angel hair pasta
Onions
Celery
Carrots
2 garlic cloves

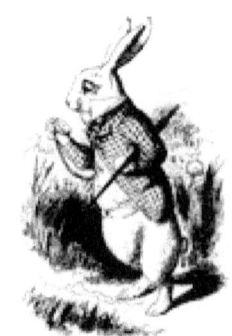

2 cups flower
Pepper
Paprika
2 cups of beef stock
1 can of tomato sauce

Instructions:
Quarter the big bunny and soak in some lightly beaten eggs. Soak for 15 minutes.

Boil some water to cook some linguini or angel hair pasta. Finely dice two cups of onions, one cup celery, and one cup carrots, two cloves of garlic and set aside. Roll the soaked bunny quarters in flour seasoned well with salt pepper paprika and garlic powder. Transfer to a hot tall-sided sauté pan with a thin coat of oil on the bottom.

Cooking the rabbit all the way through isn't necessary. Just braze it and flip it only once. Remove from pan to a plate when it has reached a nice golden brown crust. Add the chopped vegetables two cups of beef stock or broth and scrape the stuck-on food off the bottom of the pan with a spatula. Add a can of tomato sauce and then put the bunny back in the pan and cook on low heat until the rabbit is done and tender.

Plate the rabbit on top of the pasta and serve.

> *"Ewwie! That was some good rabbit! Thanks for such a great recipe! I sure enjoyed this, bouncy, tasty meat. Course I had to eat it all myself cuz the wife and kids had grown so attached to the little fella, they couldn't touch a bit of it. I told them NOT to get too attached! I'm the father, and I have to do what I think is right! I'll miss Mr. Snuggles also. Don't worry. I got my kids a new pet turkey just yesterday.*
> **-Jim (Turbo) Lufkin of Tire Fire, TN**

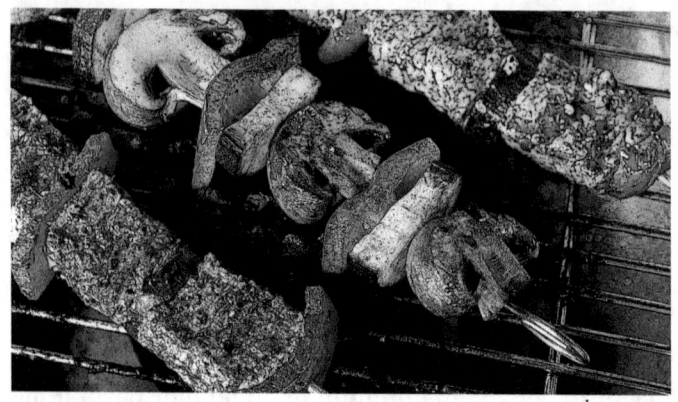
yelp

Mushroom Head Teriyaki Skewers
Gochew Grill
Truth Or Consequences, New Mexico

The "Truth" is New Mexico is cattle country. The "Consequences" is you could starve to death if you're a vegetarian living there. So if you are a vegetarian it is really good to find a good purple mushroom head to lovingly slip all the way down your throat. Fortunately, all the gobblers of the purple-headed pineapple sauce slingers can get their chew on at the legendary *Gochew Grill*.

This is a delicious meatless kabob recipe – perfect for an afternoon of backyard entertaining with friends or a late-night snack. A great night to pull out that great Sake you've been hoarding too!

Ingredients:
1 cup (packed) light brown sugar
1 cup mirin
1 cup soy sauce
1 tablespoon sesame oil
1/4 teaspoon sriracha sauce
4 large portabella mushrooms
1 fresh pineapple
1 large red onion
olive oil

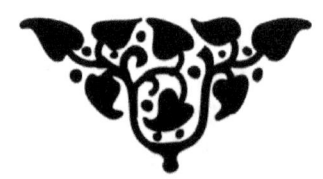

Instructions:
Core the pineapple and onion into even-sized cubes. Using a paper towel or mushroom brush remove any dirt from the mushrooms. Remove the stem, and then cut into quarters. Evenly skewer the mushrooms, pineapple, and onions.

Preheat the grill to 400 degrees. Lightly spray or drizzle olive oil on each skewer, then place on the grill. Baste with some of the teriyaki sauce. Grill until lightly browned, about 3-5 minutes.

Turn over the kabob, baste with more teriyaki and grill another 3-5 minutes until the mushrooms and onions are cooked throughout, and the pineapple is caramelized. Serve. Best with Sake and more Sake or see what Pussy says below:

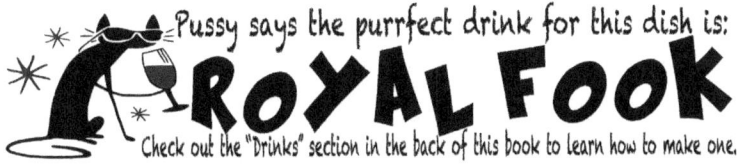

Check out the "Drinks" section in the back of this book to learn how to make one.

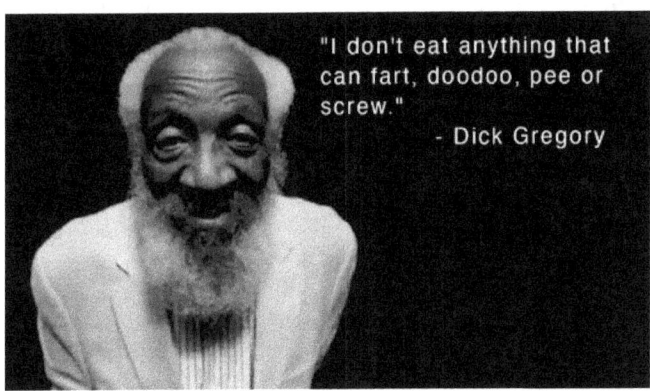

"I don't eat anything that can fart, doodoo, pee or screw."
- Dick Gregory

With all this crap they put in meat, like hormones for fast growing, antibiotics, etc... we will all go down, there's only the vegetarians that will survive - so let me give you a good piece of advice: if you want to eat some healthy meat, eat a vegetarian!
   -JeanLuc LeMoine, French humorist

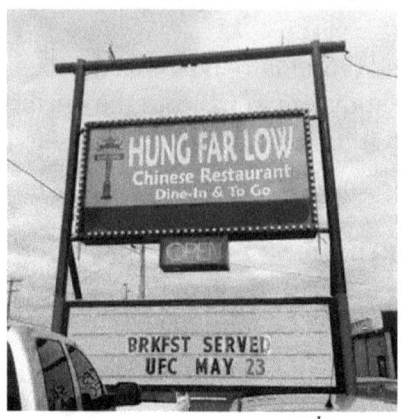
yelp

Loin Knockers With Small Onions
Hung Far Low
Mock City, Washington

The Best Baked Garlic Pork Loin Knocker recipe ever… incredibly easy, delicious, and bursting with flavors the whole family loves!

Hung Far Low Loin Knockers are an incredibly versatile dinner that tastes excellent dine in or dine out. With a ton of different preparations; with veggies, in a stir fry, salads, or even sandwiches and wraps. It is unique on its own! It will tantalite your tongue, expand your throat, and terrify your tonsils. "It's a whole watta' food."

It comes with a rib-spreader. Extra insurance of some kind is highly recommended before you dig in.

Ingredients:
1 boneless pork loin roast (3 to 4 pounds)
3 tablespoons olive oil
5 garlic cloves, minced
1 teaspoon salt
1 teaspoon each dried basil, thyme and rosemary, crushed
1/2 teaspoon Italian seasoning
1/2 teaspoon pepper
8 medium carrots, halved lengthwise
2 medium onions, quartered

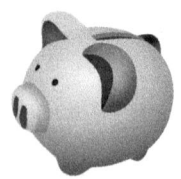

Instructions:
In a small bowl, mix oil, garlic, and seasonings; rub over roast.

Arrange carrots and onions on the bottom of a 13x9-inch baking pan. Place roast over vegetables, fat side up. Refrigerate covered for 1 hour.

Preheat oven to 475° and roast the pork for 20 minutes. Reduce oven setting to 425°. Roast 30-40 minutes longer or until the thermometer reads 145° and the vegetables are tender. Remove roast from oven; tent with foil. Let stand 20 minutes before slicing.

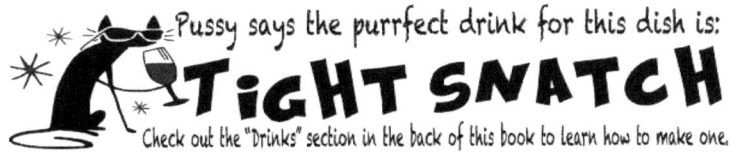

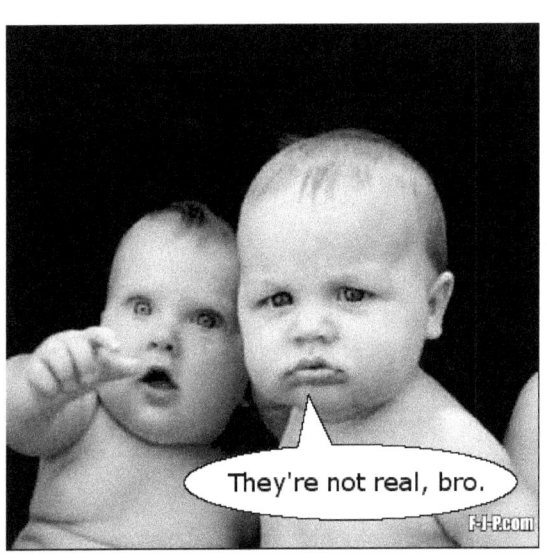

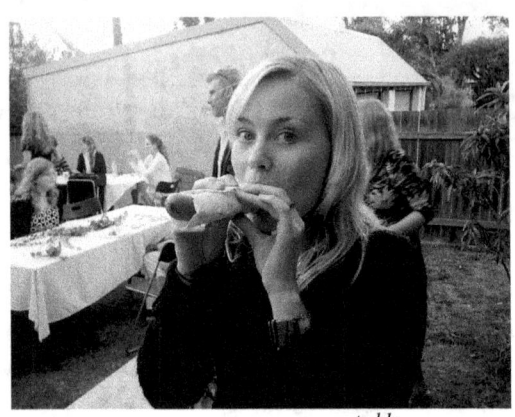
tmblr

Mr. Big's Skin Flutes
Late Night Dine Right
San Francisco, CA.

They look like a skinny version of the musical instrument. They aren't. They are just meat flutes.

You can't play music on them but, putting a big one in your mouth can really make a mouth *hummmm* with delight.

Ingredients:
1.1 lbs. of Skirt Steak
10 Corn Tortillas
1 Avocado
1 Tomato
1/4 of a Lettuce
1 Onion
2 Garlic cloves
3 Bay Leaves
1/2 cup of Mexican Cream
1/4 cup of crumbled Fresh Cheese
1 cup of Vegetable Oil
1 tablespoon of Salt

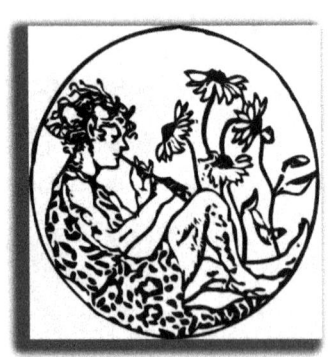

Instructions:
Cook the Skirt Steak in a pan.

Chop and add ½ onion and 2 garlic cloves and add the bay leaves and a tablespoon of Salt.

Bring a saucepan with water to a boil over high heat, then reduce it to medium heat. Add your meat and cover the saucepan. Leave your meat cooking for approximately 1 hour until it is well cooked and soft. Let it cool and then shred.

Slice 1 tomato in half. Cut lettuce into strips. Chop 1/2 onion and then set them all aside.

Heat on a griddle over medium heat 10 tortillas for about 30 seconds per each side, until they are soft. Put on each one some of the shredded skirt steaks. Roll the tortillas up and close them with some toothpicks. Eat the meat flutes quick before they soften and get all limp. No one likes a limp flute.

"I've been putting Mr. Big's Meat Flute up to my lips and enjoying them for years. You could call me a Meat Flute Virtuoso! I'm a real slob about too. I've ruined I don't know how many of my shirts with Mr. Big's Meat Flute juice. You can't get it out!

The dry cleaner recognized the Meat Flute Juice right away. Said he "I can't get dat juice outta of my own shirts! Now we eat Mr. Big's Meat Flutes and dirty up our shirts together every Friday night! Thanks Mr. Big!"
    -Dr. Tom "Self-taught" Parker

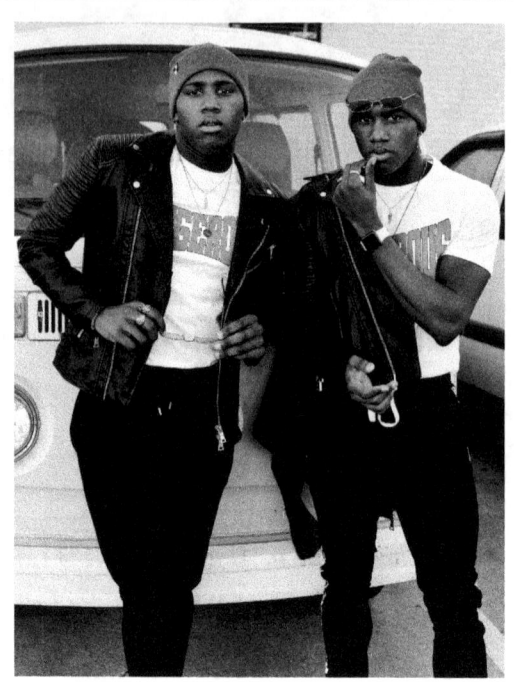

BIG JIM AND THE TWINS
CHOPS & HOPS
TWO WALLNUTS, FLORIDA

Big Jim owns this restaurant and keeps his "two twins" handy. Everyone that has ever seen Big Jim's twins say they are a couple of nuts.

Ingredients:
10 pork bratwurst links
1 stick unsalted butter
1 large onion, thinly sliced
1 bottle of beer
Mustard (optional)

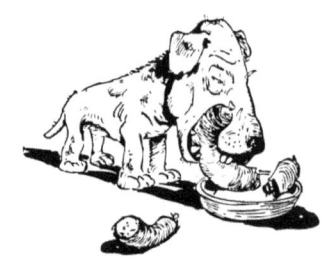

Instructions:
The hotter you get your coals going, the better the brats are going to be. When the briquettes are ready, distribute the charcoal evenly.

Place the butter in a shallow, heavy-duty aluminum foil pan on one side of the grill, and place the brats on the other side of the grill directly on the grate. When the butter melts, add the onions and the beer. Stir until the onions are soft.

Turn the brats as needed until they are nicely browned. (Don't worry about them being undercooked; they will finish cooking in the pan.) Add them to the pan, cover with aluminum foil and cook, about 15 minutes.

Remove foil and continue to cook the brat, letting the liquid in the pan reduce until it's at least halfway gone or about 15 minutes.

Serve warm with a spoonful of the juicy onions and some mustard.

Goes perfect with any sports event, especially the one's where people repetitively get hit in the face with balls.

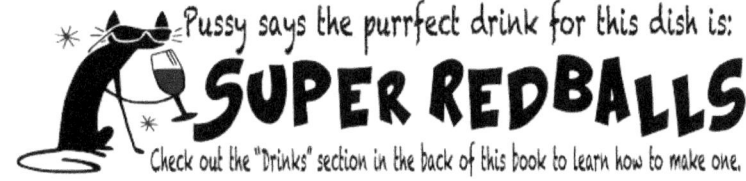

Pussy says the purrfect drink for this dish is: **SUPER REDBALLS**
Check out the "Drinks" section in the back of this book to learn how to make one.

"I was eating in a Chinese restaurant downtown. There was a dish called Mother and Child Reunion. It's chicken and eggs. And I said, I gotta use that one."
   -Paul Simon

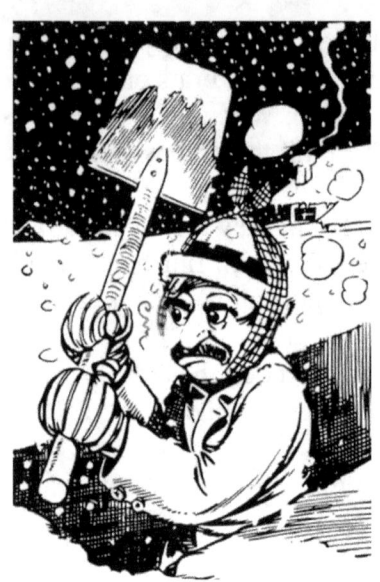

Little Willies
Two Men and a Griddle
Embarrass, MN.

The *Two Men and a Griddle* have nothing to be embarrassed about their *Little Willies*. Although very small, they still pack big taste! Some say it's the freezing cold that makes willies get so small. Others say it's 100% genetics.

Ingredients:
1 pack *Little Smokies*
Half-bottle of your favorite BBQ sauce

Instructions:
Place your Little Smokies in Crock Pot. Pour half-bottle BBQ sauce over your little Smokies.

Cook on high for 1.5 – 2 hours. Stirring occasionally

Pop a brew.

Eat them *Little Willie's* with pride!

> "My nookie days are over,
> My pilot light is out.
> What used to be my sex appeal,
> Is now my water spout.
> Time was when, on its own accord,
> From my trousers it would spring.
> But now I've got a full time job,
> To find the gosh darn thing.
> It used to be embarrassing,
> The way it would behave.
> For every single morning,
> It would stand and watch me shave.
> Now as old age approaches,
> It sure gives me the blues.
> To see it hang its little head,
> And watch me tie my shoes!!"
>
> **-Willie Nelson**

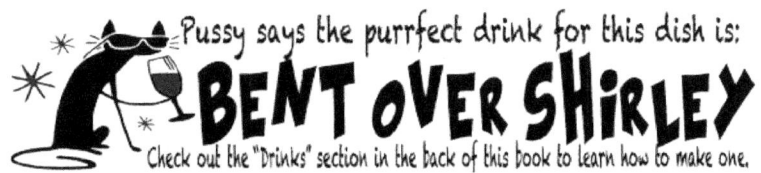

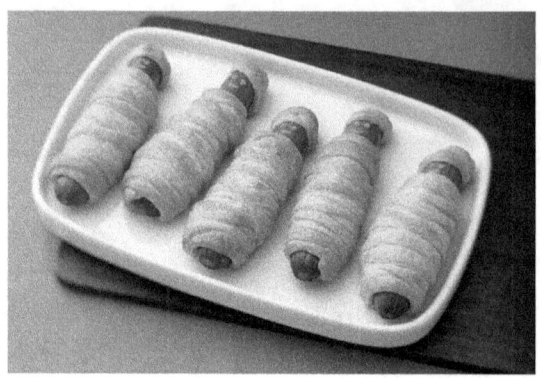
Pillsbury

WRAP THAT WEINER
THAI ME UP RESTAURANT & BREWERY PROTECTION, KS.

They love wrapping up their wieners in Protection Kansas. When Oscar Mayer sticks his wiener into the Pillsbury Doughboy at the *Thai Me Up Restaurant & Brewery,* you will find a very tasty treat in the end.

Ingredients:
1 can (8 oz) Pillsbury™ refrigerated crescent rolls
2 ½ slices American cheese, quartered
10 Oscar Mayer™ wieners
Cooking spray
Mustard or ketchup or whatever goop you love licking off a hot wiener.

Instructions:
Heat oven to 375°.

Unroll dough; separate at perforations, creating 4 rectangles. Press perforations to seal. If using dough sheet: Unroll dough; cut into 4 rectangles. With knife or kitchen scissors, cut each rectangle lengthwise into 10 pieces, making a total of 40 pieces of dough.

Cut the cheese slices into quarters (1/2 slice cheese, cut in half).

Wrap 4 pieces of dough around each hot dog and 1/4 slice of

cheese to look like "bandages," stretching dough slightly to completely cover your wiener. About 1/2 inch from one end of each wiener, separate "bandages" so wiener shows through for "face."

On an ungreased cookie sheet, place wrapped hot dogs (cheese side down); spray dough lightly with cooking spray.

Bake 13 to 17 minutes or until dough is light golden brown and wieners are hot.

With mustard, draw features on "face." What could be more fun than that?

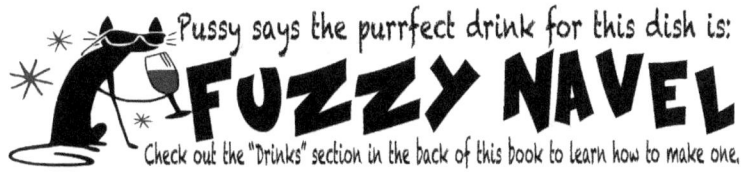

"I thought I'd shoved wieners into my mouth in every imaginable way, shape and color but no! Wrap That Wiener was fun to make and super yummy to stuff into my fur-covered face hole! Perfect for game day when all the guys come over mouths waterin' for fresh hot wiener. The hit of the day! "Go Bears!
  -Tom "Weiner Man" Chicago, Illinois

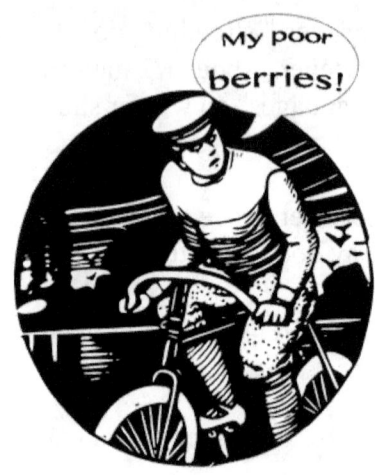

BLACK & BLUE LITTLE BERRIES YOGURT SAUCE
BLACK & BLUE BERRIES CAFÉ
SHUSHUP, WI.

This lil' dairy town is known not only for its world-renowned *Left-handed Flyswatters* and its *Mysterious Black Spotted Soup* but also for the *Black & Blue Berries Café*. Shushup is the bicycling capitol of the world.

Tell me again why in the hell do we still need that bar that runs form the handlebars to the seat?

Ingredients:
2/3 cup frozen blueberries
2/3 cup frozen blackberries
1/2 cup water
1/4 cup sugar
2 tablespoons fresh lemon juice
1 tablespoon butter
2 cups plain 2% reduced-fat Greek yogurt

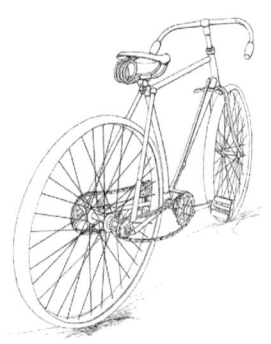

Instructions:

Combine the first 5 ingredients in a small saucepan and bring mixture to a boil.

Reduce heat to medium-low and gently boil 10 minutes or so until sauce thickens and then stir in butter.

Spoon about a 1/2 cup yogurt into each of 4 bowls and top each serving with about 1/4 cup sauce.

Serve immediately.

*"The tastiest berries are often hidden.
Do not despair if you haven't found true love.
Look under the leaves and branches of convention."*

- ***Khang Kijarro Nguyen***

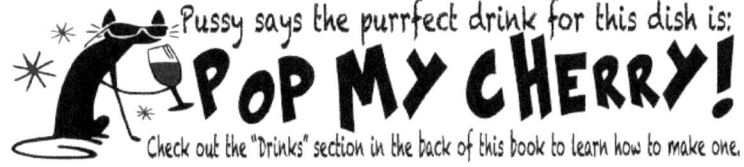

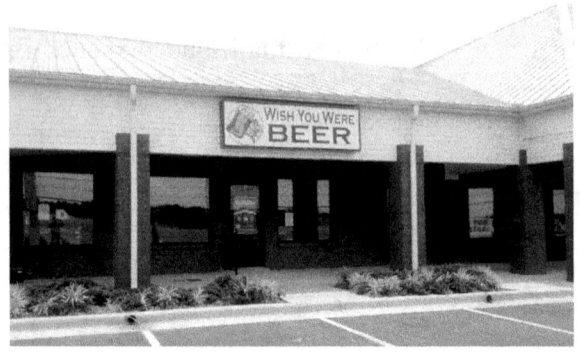

yelp

Slow-Cooker Beer Brats
Wish you were Beer
Hempstead, NY

Most of my family lives in Wisconsin. Besides the Green Bay Packers, Wisconsin is known for their beer, brats, and cheese.

In this slow cooker beer brats recipe, I am going to teach you the tricks I have learned on how to cook the most delicious crockpot beer brats and onions you will ever make!

Wisconsin natives have their own tricks to making the perfect brats. Some people cook them in beer and onions before grilling them and others grill the brats first. I grill my brats first to lock in the crispy skin.

Ingredients:
12 fresh bratwurst
2 sweet onions, sliced
4 cloves crushed garlic
4 tablespoons butter
1/2 teaspoon salt
1/2 teaspoon pepper
3 bottles of crappy beer

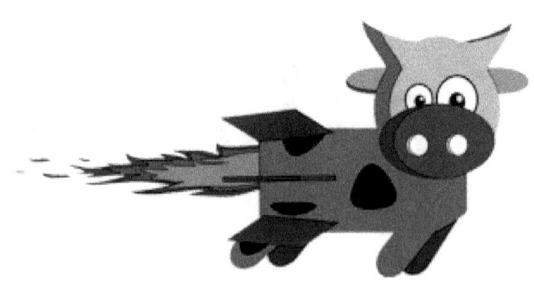

Instructions:

In 10-inch nonstick skillet, cook bratwurst over medium-high heat, frequently turning, just until the outsides are brown.

Place in the slow cooker. Top with onion slices, garlic, butter, salt, and pepper. Pour in a crappy beer like PBR. Cover and cook on High heat setting 4 hours or Low heat setting 7 to 8 hours.

Eat and share your wieners.

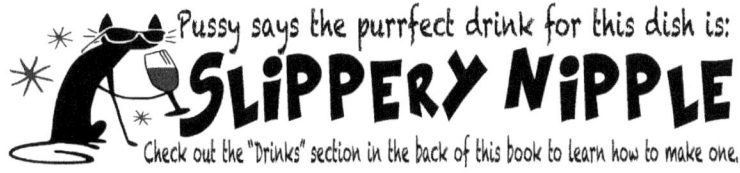

Pussy says the purrfect drink for this dish is: **SLIPPERY NIPPLE**
Check out the "Drinks" section in the back of this book to learn how to make one.

"In Pakistan, anti-American protesters set a Kentucky Fried Chicken restaurant on fire. The protesters mistakenly thought they were attacking high-ranking U.S. military official Colonel Sanders."
   -Jimmy Fallon

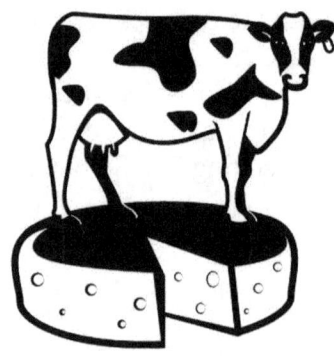

Beer Cheese Beer Beefy Brats and Beer
Bacon Bros. Diner
Redwing MN.

The boys at *Bacon Brothers Diner* love der Beer Cheese Beer Beefy Brats, and Beer just love their cheesy beer brats. They like to stick them in a bun and get them all cheesy. Some like to dip them in cheese and lick them too.

Ingredients:
Beefy Brats
Beer
Cheese
Beer
Beer
Beer

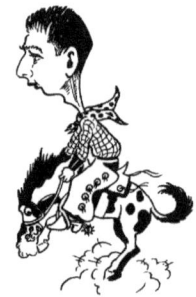

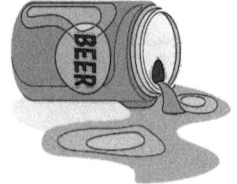

Instructions:

Add beer and brats to sauce pan. Cook on medium-high heat for 10-15 minutes or about a quarter of play depending on commercials and injuries.

Place brats on the grill and cook until done. 10 to15 min. or right around half time.

With 1 cup of beer in the pot, add cream cheese and cheddar. Stir during the half-time report or until cheese is mixed.

Add the cheese mixture on top of the beer brats.

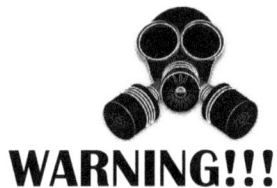

WARNING!!!

Beefy Brats + Cheeses + Beers = Big toots from the boot.
(Keep your friends and family safe. ...open a window or three!)

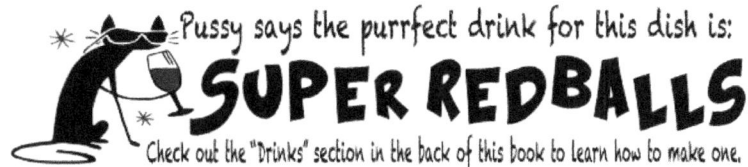

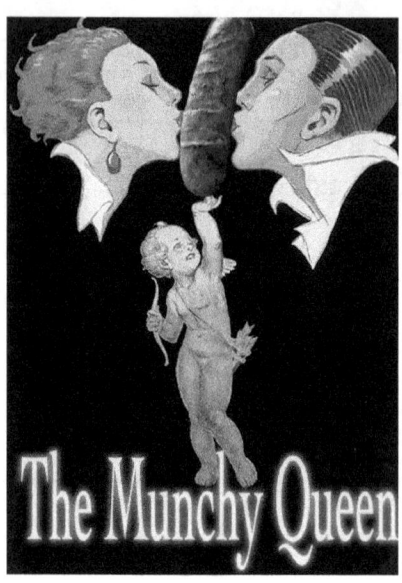

Wrapped Mini-wieners
The Munchy Queen
Plano, Texas

Down in Plain O Texas, they wrap their mini-wieners up in their "Wicked Moon Crescent Rolls." For the big wieners, they just use a loaf of bread.

You can smell this place from miles off and see the grey wiener smoke trailing up into the never-ending Texas sky. Established in 1937. *The Munchy Queen* has been sucking down wieners for so long they had been granted a Texas State Historical Landmark plaque in 1997. Worth seeing. Really!

Ingredients:
48 cocktail-size smoked link sausages or hot dogs. Whatever you like in yer mouth best.

2 cans refrigerated crescent rolls

Instructions:
Place sausage on the shortest side of each triangle and roll up each weenie in its own dough triangle. Lay them all out on an ungreased cookie sheet. Leave room in between to allow for wiener/dough expansion while cooking.

Bake 12 to 15 minutes or until golden brown. Immediately remove from the cookie sheet. Serve warm.

Wanna get fancy? Layout some dips like mustard, catsup, and my favorite ranch dressing.

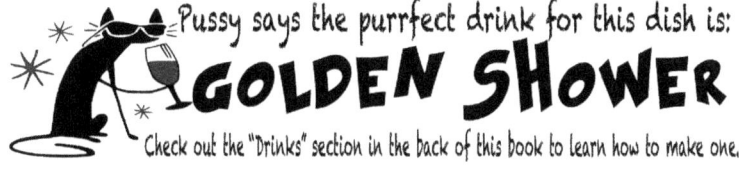

Check out the "Drinks" section in the back of this book to learn how to make one.

"I make but no can stop eat! I eat many little wiener in row. Dog watch me eat wiener and he cry and cry. Dog want eat little wiener too. I say No! Little wiener not for little dog! Little wiener only for big owner of dog like me!"
-Dong Hung Lo of Mosquito Bay FL

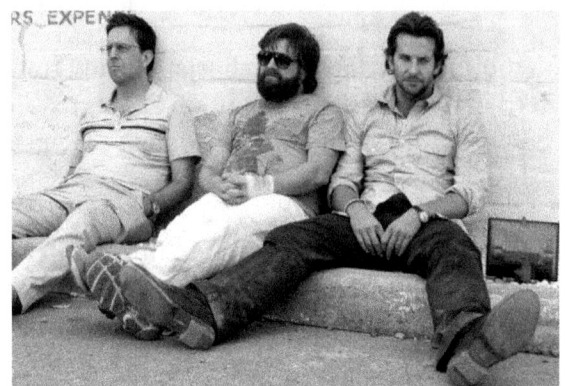
Legendary Pictures

BITE SIZE WHISKEY WIENERS
HANGOVER CURE
ACCIDENT, MARYLAND

I once made these at a sausage party of mine. Yes even though I am a girl I do really enjoy a good sausage party.

The Bite Size Whisky Wieners were by far the most popular snack of the evening. They were more popular then the large hot dogs. Also by far they were the easiest to make.

They've got whiskey in the wieners, they take two minutes to put together, they're eaten with toothpicks, and everybody except the snootiest of the snoots loves them.

By the way, even after several hours of slow-cooking, the whiskey aroma can still be quite powerful. And of course, the best thing to pair whiskey wieners with is... whiskey.

I've heard that some people choose to throw alliteration to the wind and serve Tequila Wieners, but that sounds just a bit too wild for me.

WARNING!
Though some people might think that the alcohol gets cooked off in dishes like this. I am happy to report it does <u>not</u>! Perhaps this is how "Accident," Maryland got its name.

Ingredients:
1 pound cocktail franks (or mini smoked sausages)
1/2 cup ketchup
1/2 cup brown sugar (packed, light or dark)
1/4 teaspoon *Worcestershire* sauce
1/2 cup barbecue sauce
3 to 116 tablespoons of bourbon (to taste)

Instructions:
In a slow-cooker, combine the ketchup, brown sugar, Worcestershire sauce, barbecue sauce, and bourbon. Stir to blend thoroughly. Did I mention the bourbon?

Add the cocktail franks or mini smoked sausages to the sauce and stir to coat. Cover the pot and cook on high for 1 hour; remove the lid and cook on low for 1 hour longer.

Keep the setting on low or switch it to warm and serve the cocktail franks hot from the slow cooker. Just like mom used to.

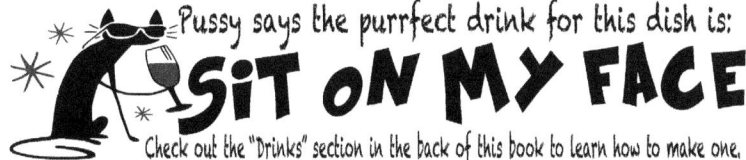

Pussy says the purrfect drink for this dish is: SIT ON MY FACE
Check out the "Drinks" section in the back of this book to learn how to make one.

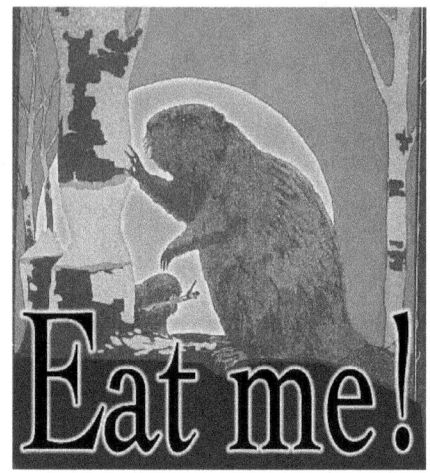

BEAVER

Everyone loves to eat some sweet, tasty beaver every now and then.

What's better than munching on beaver until the sweet juices squirt out dripping down our trembling chins?

Perfect with any clam, candles and red wine.

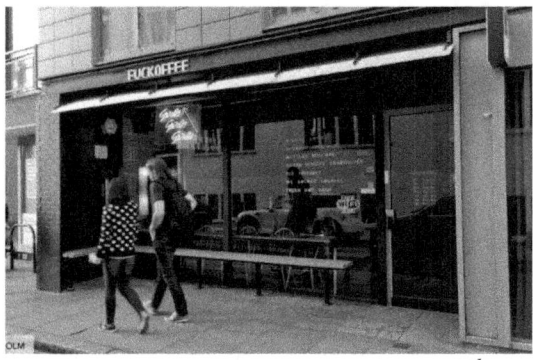
yelp

Shaved Asian Beavers
Fuckoffee
Cut And Shoot, Texas

Nothing is tastier then eating *Shaved Asian Beavers* at *Fuckoffee!*

I like to lick mine for hours on end to make it really last. I think the tail might be my favorite part.

Try marinating it in olive oil and garlic sauce. The great thing about that sauce is you can use it on any meat you want to make it sweet.

Ingredients:
1/2 cup soy sauce
1/2 cup olive oil
6 cloves garlic

Instructions:
Shave your beaver.

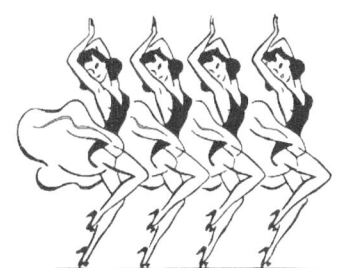

Rinse your beaver and pat your beaver dry. Some prefer to dry their beaver with a hairdryer, personally I like blowing on it myself so I don't burn it.

After you are done drying your beaver put it in a sealable plastic bag with the crushed garlic marinade. Leave the Marinade on your beaver for six hours. Rub, poke and pat it to move the juices around whenever you feel the urge. I usually throw on a disco record and crank it up.

"Shake, Shake, Shake... Shake, Shake, Shake... Shake Your Booty... Shake Your Booty..."

Preheat your oven to 500 degrees.

Put clarified butter in a cast iron skillet and heat it up until smoking and throw your beaver in there. Put the skillet into your oven at 500 degrees for 5 minutes, then let it rest outside the oven for ten minutes.

I had been worried that the soy and garlic would overpower the natural beaver juice's. If I'm going to eat beaver, I don't want sauces to disguise the delicate taste. But in reality, it complimented the taste of the beaver and teased out its gaminess.

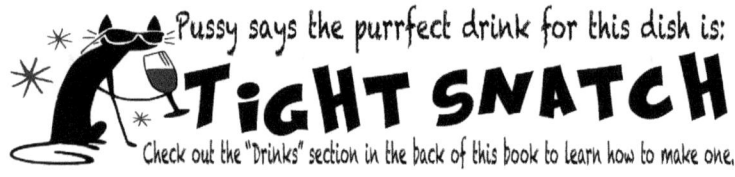

"Some people ask the secret of our long marriage. We take time to go to a restaurant two times a week. A little candlelight, dinner, soft music, and dancing. She goes Tuesdays, I go Fridays."
    -Henry Youngman

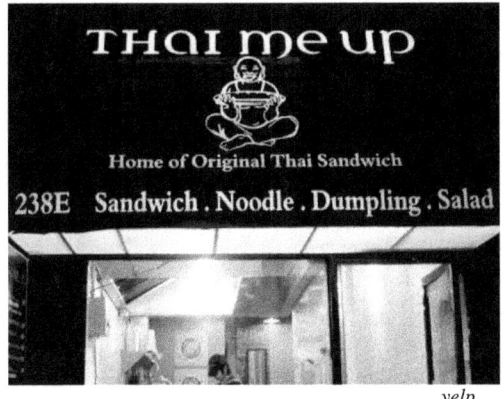
yelp

S&M's Tender Beaver
Thai Me Up
Frustrated, Oklahoma

Sam and Mary's famous recipe for beaver tenderloin.

This recipe will be especially enjoyed by those who like to tie their meat up before eating it. Sam and Mary or "S&M" as the locals call them will tie your beaver up for you if you want!

Ingredients:
1 whole beaver tenderloin, trimmed of all visible fat. You guessed it, shave that beaver like you mean it!
Kosher salt
2 teaspoons sugar
1/2 cup tri-color peppercorns, crushed with a rolling pin
1 stick butter
2 cloves garlic, crushed

Instructions:
Preheat the oven to 475 degrees.

Tie your beaver up with a small rope or twine. Rub into the soft exposed flesh some fresh ground pepper, kosher salt and some hot jalapeno juice if you like it spicy. Put clarified butter in a cast iron skillet and heat it up until smoking.

Put the skillet into your oven for 8 minutes or longer depending on the size of your beaver then let your beaver relax outside the oven for 10 minutes covered with aluminum foil.

Now place your meat on a roasting rack. Sprinkle it generously with kosher salt and sugar, which will deepen the savory flavors.

Press the crushed peppercorns all over the surface of the meat. Insert a meat thermometer and place in the oven until the beef registers 120 to 125 degrees for medium-rare/rare. Cook 20 to 25 minutes.

While the meat is roasting, melt the butter with the garlic in a small skillet, and allow the butter to slightly brown. Remove the garlic and discard.

Remove the meat when it's done and pour the garlic butter over gently (it should sizzle when it hits the meat). Cover the meat loosely with foil and allow your beaver to rest for 10 minutes before slicing. It is so much more fun when everyone eats beaver together.

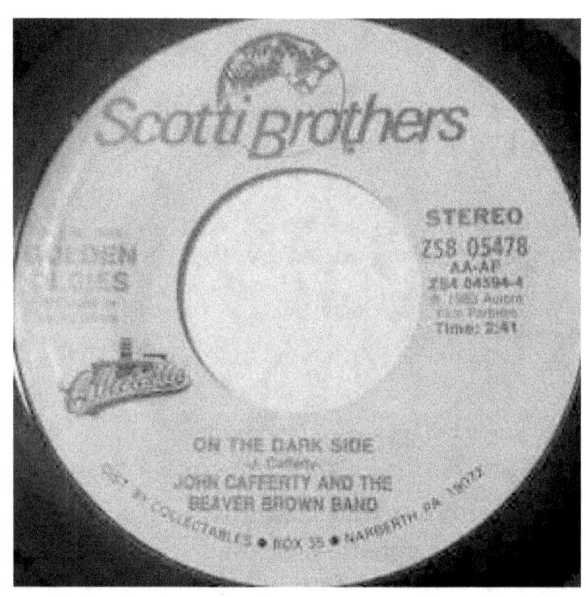

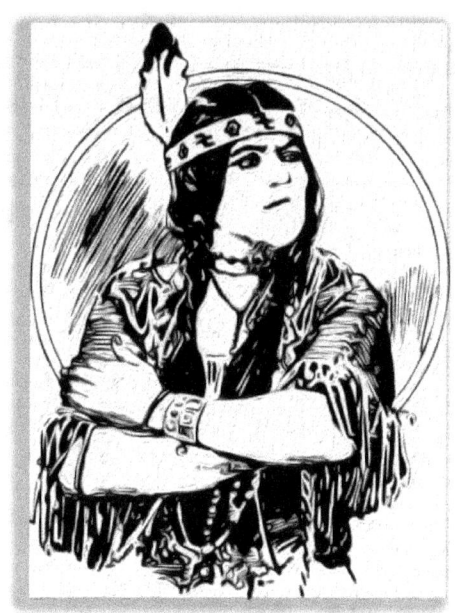
One Drunk Beaver

ONE DRUNK BEAVER
CUSTARDS LAST STAND
SOMEFIELD SD.

This dish from *Custard's Last Stand* is named after One Drunk Beaver. She was a very strong and brave Indian woman who famously whooped it up on white men whenever she drank alcohol.

> *I'll remember the first time I ate One Drunk Beaver. The beaver was much easier to acquire and eat then I thought. All it took was one good shot and a couple of beers. But she really was one tough, hairy beaver!*
> **-Wyatt Earp,** *Hole in The Wall Gang*

Ingredients:
1 Beaver Tail (the bigger the better)

Instructions:
Hold your beaver tail over an open flame until all the rough skin blisters and loosens. You never want to eat a beaver that has skin blisters on it or loose skin.

Remove from heat and immediately pour a bottle of whiskey over it and boom! *One Drunk Beaver Tail!*

When cool, peel off skin. Roast over coals or simmer until tender then eat it all night long.

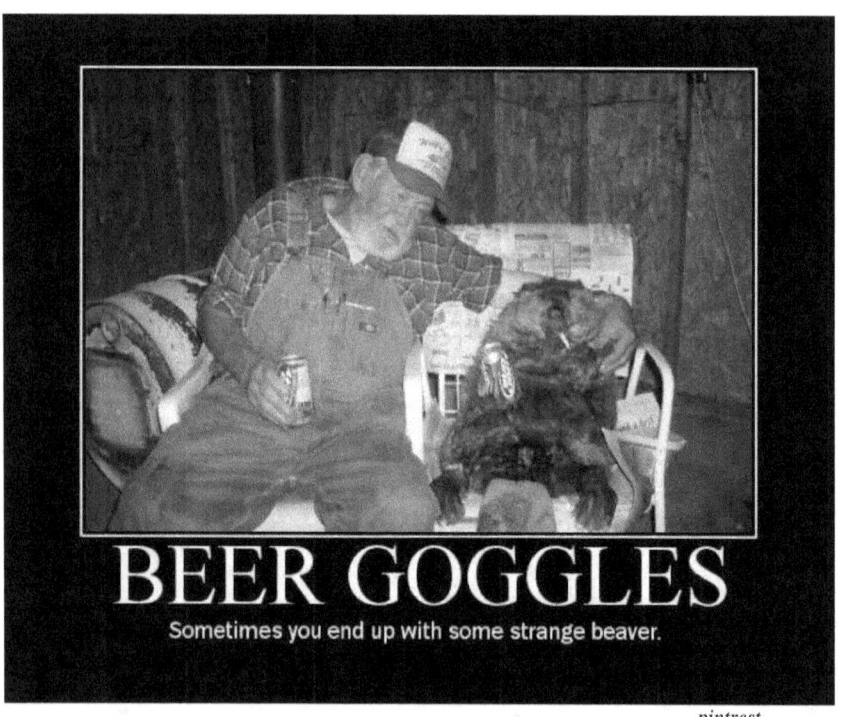

pintrest

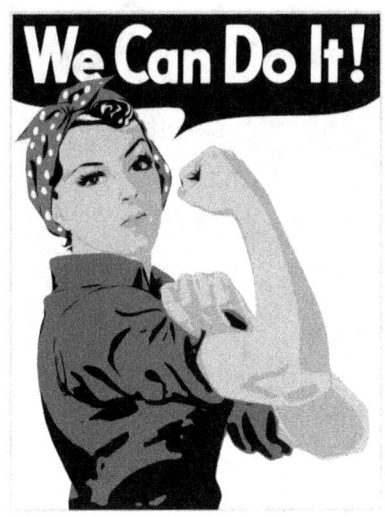

CAN DO BEAVER
DECADENT DESIRE
LAS VEGAS, NEVADA

Rosie the Riveter was the star of a campaign aimed at recruiting female workers for the defense industries during World War II. She became perhaps the most iconic image of all women during that time when men were so scarce. These are the "Rosie's" that took over doing everything the men were doing at home and at work before they left for war. Rosies knew how to keep the home fires burning. They also made them hot and steamy at night.

The Rosie's at *Decadent Desire* know how to treat a beaver right because they have one, and you can get it done right for once.

Here's to all the *Can Do Beaver* women of the world and thank you for keeping all the girls happy at home and those *Decadent Desires* churning while all the men were away at war.

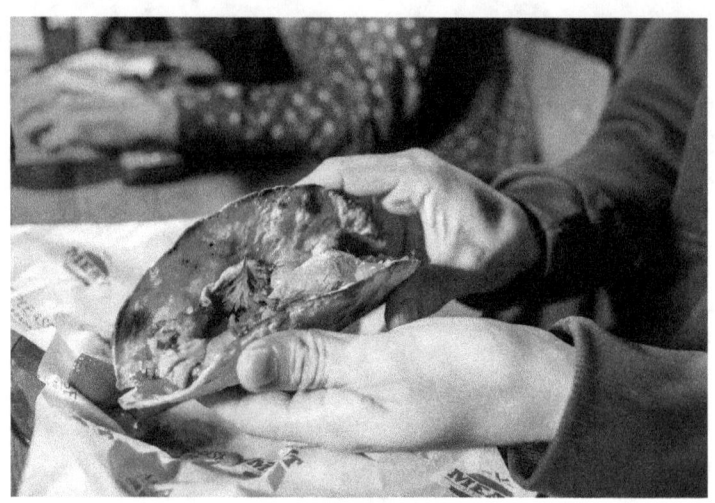

Rosie's Giant Pink Corn Taco & White Cream Sauce
The Pink Taco Van
South Side Los Angeles, CA.

Rosie is defiantly a "Can Do Beaver" type gal that knows how to eat beaver really well. But sometimes she prefers to put big hunks of beef in her taco.

In South L.A. where Rosie sells her *Giant Pink Taco & White Cream Sauce* out on the street is in a bad neighborhood. Sure it got its gangs, drug problems, and police brutality, but *The Pink Taco Van* is worth the risk even if you have to make an occasional run from it.

These are the best pink tacos on Earth! You can't be angry with a Rosie's Pink Taco flopping around in your mouth and her special white sauce runnin' down your chin. It's a beautiful thing.

Ingredients:
1 lb flank or skirt steak
12 pink corn tortillas

For the Marinade

3 limes, juiced
1 orange, juiced
¼ C. oil (I used olive oil)
5-6 cloves garlic, minced
Sour Cream
½ jalapeño, finely chopped (remove vien and seeds if you don't want it too spicy)
1 tsp. cumin
½ tsp. chile powder (I like chipotle chili powder)
½ tsp. oregano
½ tsp. salt
several grinds of fresh black pepper
¾ C. chopped fresh cilantro (about a large handful)
Garnish - choose what you like
chopped cilantro
diced white onions (grilled onions would be yummy too!)
lime wedges
avocado slices
pico de gallo
crumbled Cotija cheese or Queso Fresco

Instructions:
Combine marinade ingredients in small bowl and mix well. Put steak and marinade in zip lock bag and let steak marinate for a few hours.

Remove steak from marinade. Grill steak to desired doneness.

Remove from grill and let your steak rest a bit, then slice against grain into thin strips.

Fill your warmed pink corn tortillas with some steak, top with additional cilantro, onions, sour cream and squeeze of lime.

For a more non-traditional street taco add other toppings like avocado, cheese or pico de gallo. If you want more spice top it with your favorite hot sauce.

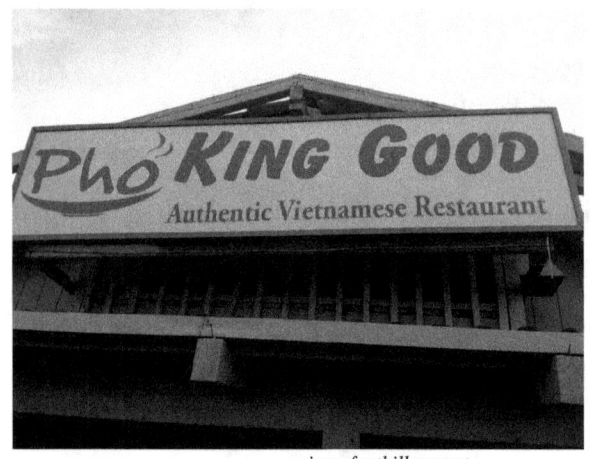
sierrafoothillsreport

Pho King Beaver Bangers
Pho King Good Noodles
Truth or Consequences, NM.

Everyone loves Pho King Beaver. Eating a fresh beaver can be a *Pho King* challenge in such a small town like *Truth or Consequences*. Most of the beaver there has Pho King already been eaten so fresh beaver has to be imported. Since there is no airport, it actually has to be Pho King parachuted in!

Pho King Good Noodles are serious when it comes to their beaver freshness! They have the freshest *Pho King Beaver Bangers* in town. One Pho King Beaver Banger and you will defiantly get a Pho King bad case of Beaver Pho King Fever.

Ingredients:
1 cup white vinegar
1 large can crushed, diced, or whole tomatoes and their juice
2 heaping tablespoons kosher salt
2 cups beef or chicken stock
Pasta Sprinkle

Instructions:
Put the brine in a large sealable bag along with your Pho King beaver and let it sit for at least two hours or more. This is a great time to get caught up on some TV.

Maybe there's a good Pho King documentary about eating Pho King beaver. If not there's plenty of beaver eating and Pho King action to be seen on some websites.

Remember, the longer you keep that beaver wet, the more, the tastier it will become in the Pho King end. Take your time. Make it last!

Using forwards and backward strokes, push your juices in and around your beaver as much as you can. If you're having trouble try putting on a favorite record and dimming the lights a little. In an emergency …think of baseball. When done, remove your meat, rinse it, and pat it dry with a towel. You know like back in high school.

Put 2 cups of beef or chicken or beef stock depending on if you like your Pho King beaver tasting like Pho King chicken or beef. Or you could just eat it with its very own great, musky taste.

Season with a teaspoon of "Pasta Sprinkle."

The longer you let your Pho King beaver cook, the more tender it will be. You can cook your meat on high for 4 hours or on the low setting for 8 hours.

When done, you can pull that hot beaver apart with your fingers and enjoy watching your friends and Pho King eat it with your Pho King favorite hot sauce.

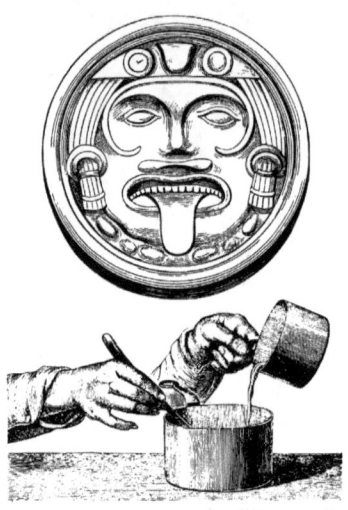

Rubs, Sauces, Stews & Soups

Basically, a rub is a mixture of spices and herbs that are applied directly to meats before cooking.

Many chefs prefer dry rubs for grilling because they won't burn, which also makes them perfect for meats that require long cooking times, like briskets and ribs.

Your Rubing Tips

Just like any form of cooking, there are some general tips and tricks that will make your first meat rub a lot easier:

Use one to two tablespoons of a dry rub for each pound of meat.

Rubs using lemon juice or vinegar also change the food's texture because acids cure meat.

After applying a rub, wrap the meat in plastic and place it in the refrigerator before cooking. This will allow the meat time to absorb the flavor from the various spices. A plastic zipper bag is great for this.

Get a head start by freezing meat after applying a rub. Just thaw and enjoy at a later time.

Dry rubs can be stored for a few months, but don't try to use the mix beyond that. Make a fresh batch.

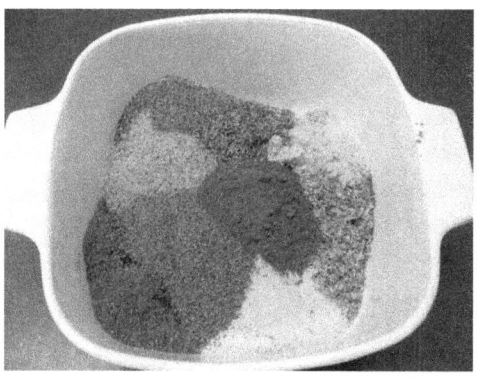

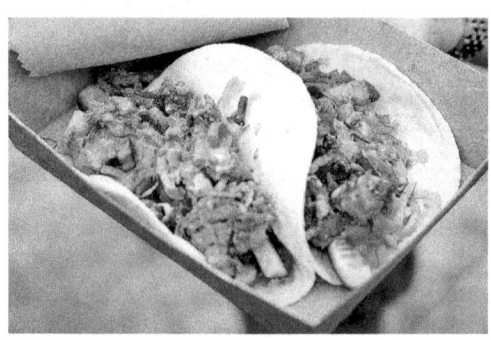

Rub One Out On Your Street Tacos
Burrito Belly
Hippo, Kentucky

Use this recipe to rub your meat out with and then fill up your *Burrito Belly* with street tacos.

Ingredients:
1 tsp each pepper, garlic, onion, thyme, smoked paprika
2 tsp rosemary
3 tsp Demi glaze
1/2 tsp sugar
1/8 tsp red pepper

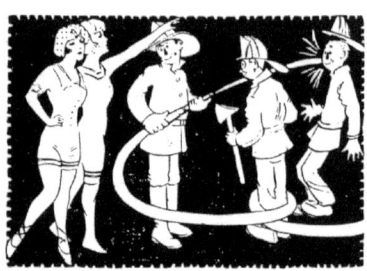

Instructions:
Combine the ingredients into a bowl to make a paste made with a bit of water.

"I went to a restaurant with the kids. The hostess said, 'How cute. Are these your kids?' I said, 'Nope. I am a representative for Trojan. These are customer complaints.'"
    -*Author Unknown*

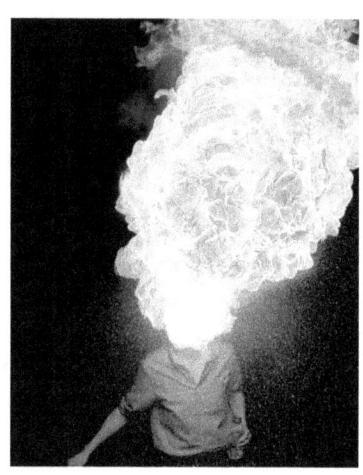

"I'M ON A DRY RUB TO HELL!" (SING IT!)
UNCLE TONY'S HOUSE
CLEVELAND, OHIO

For all those Red Hot Chili Heads out there who like to rub their meat totally dry! I really first got my hands on this around high school tore it up in junior college.

I was rubbing my meat morning noon and night. ...and sometimes twice at night. You can do it too.
   –Uncle Tony

Ingredients:
2tsp Kosher Salt
2tsp Ancho Chile Powder
1tsp Chipotle Powder
1tsp Oregano, Mexican is preferred
1tsp Gran Garlic
1tsp Gran Onion
1tsp Black Pepper
1tsp Cayenne
1-2tsp Gnd. Cumin

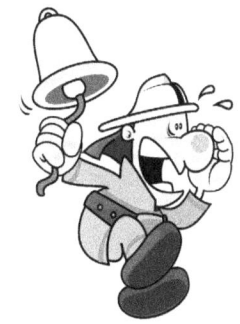

1tsp Cocoa Powder
½tsp Cinnamon

Optional:
2 tsp Turbinado Sugar (Sugar in the Raw)

Instructions:
Place in bowel with cover and shake

WARNING! This stuff is hot!!! Beyond full-flavored with a touch of smokiness. Adjust the heat to your taste by playing with the amount of black pepper, chipotle, and cayenne powders. Reduce to 1tsp. for some bite but less heat.

To really make this stuff "Hells Bells" toss in a batch of Chili, leave out the Sugar. Use on Pork, Brisket, or even just Hamburger to really get things fired up!

Makes 3/4 to 1cup of Rub.

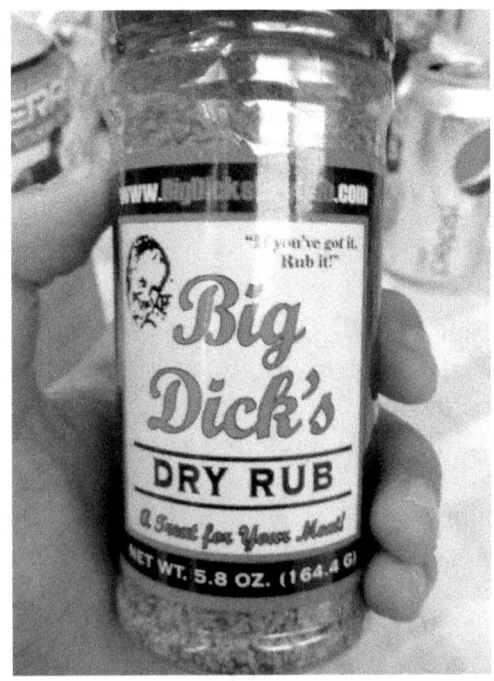

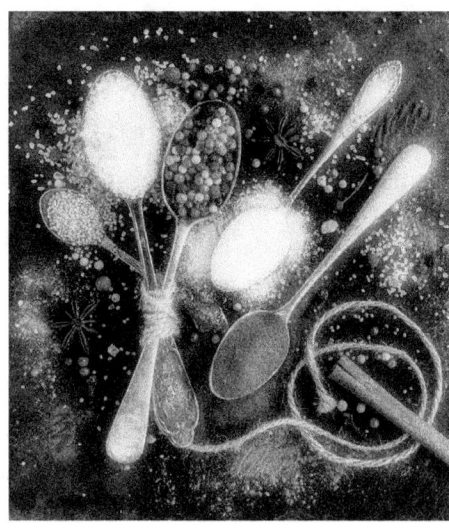

Turbo's Coffee Bean Rub
Barnyard Breakfast Diner & Automat
Chicken, Alaska

This stuff makes all meat taste something special! Now *Chicken, Alaska* is rural, to say the least. So much so that there's a parade every month when the mail comes in by dog-team. The party goes long into the night, and there's always plenty of *Turbo's Coffee Bean Rub* to keep it going.

Ingredients:
½ C Sugar in the Raw (Turbinado)
2T Sweet Paprika (Hungarian)
2T Fine Ground Coffee
1T Kosher Salt
1T Chili Powder (contains some Cumin and Oregano) Ancho Chile is same without cumin, oregano etc.
1T Granulated Garlic
1T Granulated Onion
1T Black Pepper, more if you like
1tsp Ground Coriander
1tsp Ground Dill Seed
1/2tsp Grnd. Allspice

Instructions:

Cayenne or chipotle powder to taste. Start with 1/2tsp and go up from there.

Combine the ingredients into a bowl with a bit of water to make it all a pasty.

Great on just about anything. And I do mean anything including beaver and cock!

WARNING! Be sure to wash hands of all pepper before handling your raw meat. Trust me on this one!

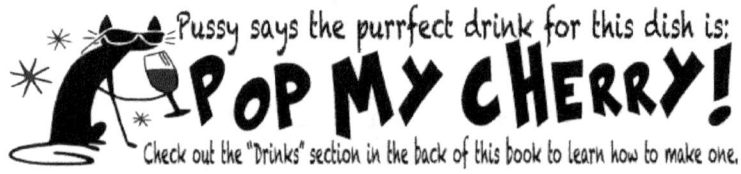

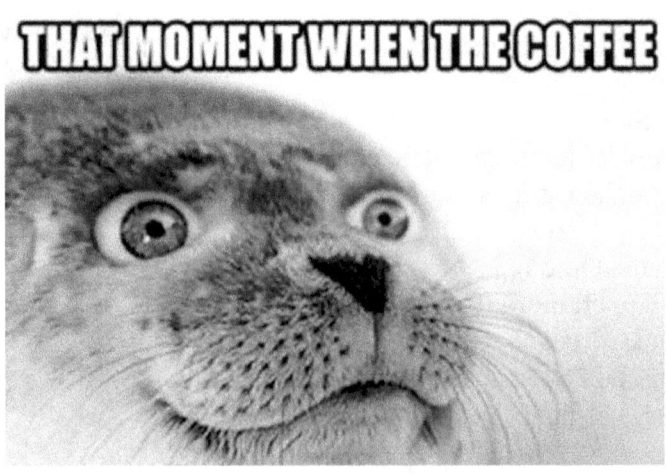

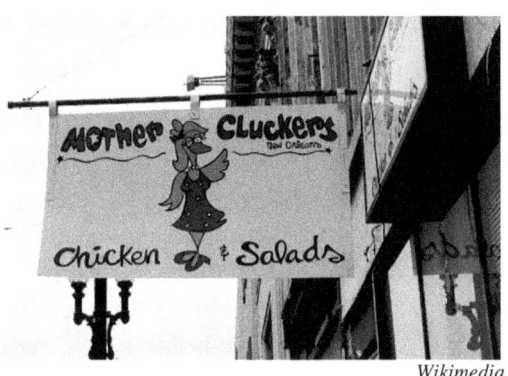
Wikimedia

Ewe Rub, I Rub, We Rub
Mother Cluckers
Hazard, Nebraska

The most significant hazard in Hazard is sheep. They get into the road and cause havoc. One wrong ewe turn and poof! Cotton balls everywhere!

All the people of Hazard care for their sheep. The town motto: "We Love Our Sheep. …don't Ewe?" At *Mother Cluckers* they have their unique own unique way of rubbing their lamb the right way.

Ingredients:
2 tsp Turbinado Sugar
2 tsp Kosher Salt
2 tsp Black Peppercorns
1 tsp Coriander Seed
1 tsp Dill Seed
1 tsp Dry Minced Onion
1 tsp Dry Minced Garlic
1 tsp Dry Lemon Peel (optional)
1 tsp Allspice Berries
1 tsp Dry Thyme Leaves
3 Bay Leaves, crumbled
1-2ea Dry Whole Chipotle Chiles, stems and seeds removed or 1tsp Chipotle Powder.
Add Cayenne if more heat is desired.

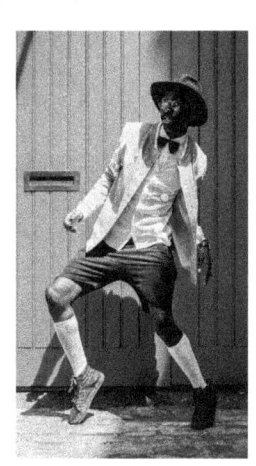

Instructions:

All Spices are whole and are toasted in a dry pan over medium heat until fragrant, 1-2 minutes. The garlic and onion do not need to be toasted.

Let the spices cool then grind in a cheapo coffee grinder until slightly less than coarse. Mix with the salt and sugar. Store in an air tight container. Makes about a half cup. Be sure to make plenty cuz folks love it!

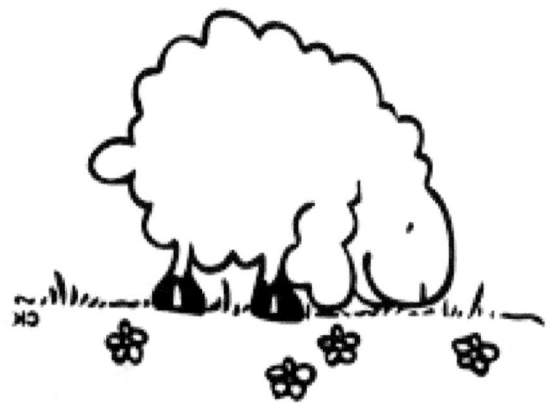

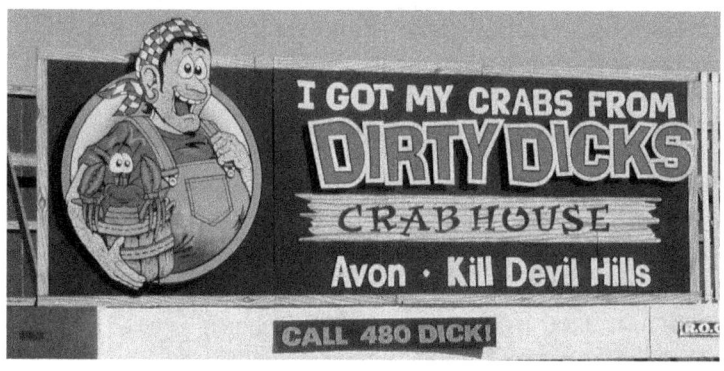

Dirty Dick's! (Rub Sauce)
Dirty Dick's Crab House
St. Petersburg, FL.

I got my crabs from Dirty Dick's, and so did my son. My husband never got the crabs and always went for the lobster. Like my husband, my daughter also does not like to get the crabs either.

My entire family gets off on Dirty Dick's. My daughter enjoys all the rubs she can get from Dirty Dick's. So now she just takes a nice rub or two home with her so she can rub any meat anytime she wants.

She really does rub all the meat she can get her hands on. My son really likes it when she rubs his meat at home. She does my husband's meat, the neighbors, and has even rubbed the postman's meat. A few years ago, she tried to rub the woman's across the street meat. We found out that she did not like Dirty Dick's so that just means more rubs for the rest of the neighborhood.

A few years ago she went to a football game, and at a tailgate party, she told me she rubbed allot of Dirty Dick's right there in the back seat of her car. Another time she took Dirty Dick's on vacation with her and rubbed everyone's meat in the hotel. She also once tried to rub the dog's meat, but he did not like it.

There is just something about the taste of Dirty Dick's that just gets her going.

WARNING! After a rubbing session with *Dirty Dicks*, you may want to wash your hands before you go to the bathroom. It is difficult to get *Dirty Dicks* off your genitals using just a sink.

Ingredients:
4 tablespoons butter
1 medium onion, chopped fine
½ red bell pepper, diced
2 tablespoons minced fresh garlic
1/4 cup Dirty Dick's Hot Pepper Sauce
3 cups ketchup
½ cup molasses
¼ cup grainy mustard
3 tablespoons balsamic vinegar
½ cup brown sugar
3 tablespoons Worcestershire sauce
juice of 1 lemon
salt and pepper to taste

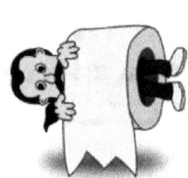

Remember what goes in must come out!

Be ready for some heavy alone time!

Instructions:
Melt butter in a saucepan, and add onion, garlic, and peppers. Sauté until onions are soft. Add the rest of the ingredients and simmer one for two hours.

Use the sauce on chicken, pork ribs, brisket or just about any meat you'd love to put into your mouth!!!

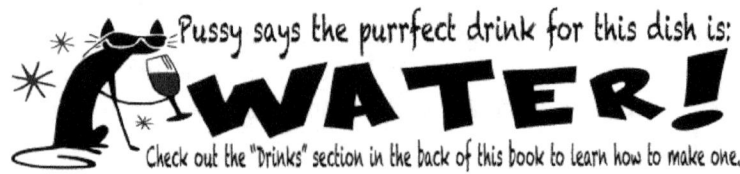

Pussy says the purrfect drink for this dish is: **WATER!** Check out the "Drinks" section in the back of this book to learn how to make one.

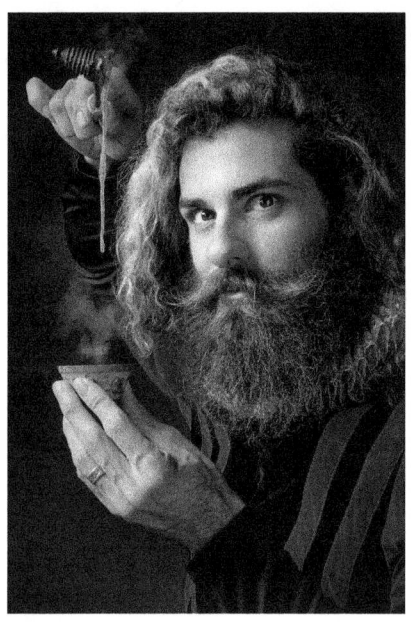

Peter's Thick White Sauce
Filled of dreams
Intercourse, PA.

Smack dab in the middle of Amish country, folks wagon in from counties near and far to get a taste of Peter's White Sauce at *Filled of Dreams*. Peter's White Sauce is something you'll be tempted to wipe off your beard, but you will leave it on there to enjoy it again for later.

You will never eat a plain white wiener again without thinking about *Peter's Thick White Sauce*!

Ingredients:
 3 tablespoons butter or margarine
 1/4 cup all-purpose flour
 1 cup milk
 1/4 teaspoon salt

Instructions:
Melt butter in a heavy saucepan over low heat; add flour, stirring until smooth. Cook for 1 minute, stirring constantly.

Gradually add milk; cook over medium heat, stirring constantly, until sauce is thickened and bubbly. Stir in salt. Did you remember to stir?

Bubbly white and thick? It's ready to be rubbed onto anyone's meat! But hang on it's going to be a wild ride right in your mouth ...at least until you swallow!

Fun for all involved!

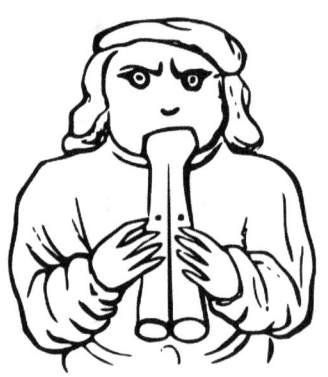

"My friends and I have contests to see who can eat the most amount of Peter's White Sauce. It sure gets messy with white souse shooting everywhere! We film it and put it up on all our pages. People love watching it in slow-motion for some reason and we don't know why." Wink!

-Josey (white sauce expert) Hillebrant

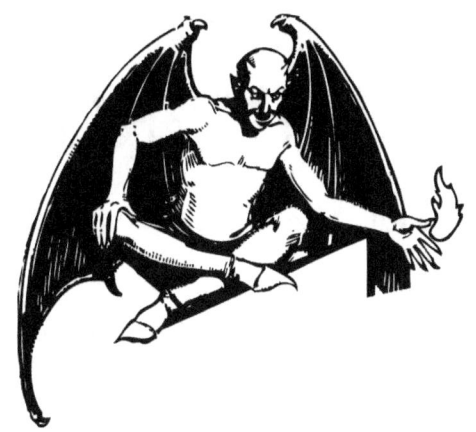

Who's Your Daddy?! Slap Sauce
Nacho Daddy's Grill
Knockemstiff, Ohio

The name says it all!

Ingredients:
20 Peppers (Fresno, Cayenne, Jalapeno) of your choice
1 1/2 cups vinegar (I used white)
1/2 tsp salt
3 tsp minced fresh garlic
1 pair Nitrate gloves
1 pair of googles
1 medium sauce pan that you can toss in a dumpster somewhere outside the city limits when your finished.

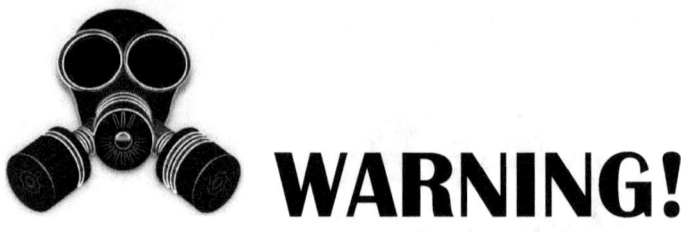

WARNING!

You might be working with crazy hot peppers! Don't get this stuff in your eyes if you want to keep 'em!

If you plan on having children wear gloves for your own protection as well as the future of mankind.

Oils from the peppers can rub off onto your hands without you even knowing it! Don't rub your eyes or next thing you know you're getting a free dog, a white cane and free passes on the bus. You've been warned!

Instructions:
Wash your peppers and cut the tops off of your peppers and slice in half lengthwise.

Pour the vinegar into a saucepan/pot, add peppers, salt, and garlic. Bring to a boil and reduce heat to a low boil until peppers are soft (about 10 minutes).

Pour everything into your blender, including peppers and vinegar. Blend it (seeds and all) until liquefied.

Add additional heat if desired. If you like it stupid hot, add a habanero remix and taste test. Have a big cold drink close by and a phone to call 911!

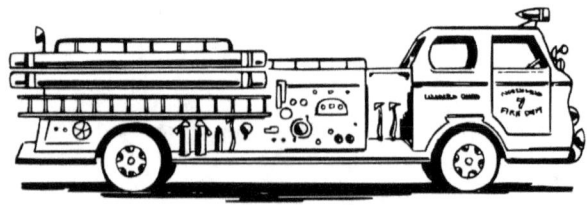

Cuz' I'm Your Mother and I said so!!
(Slap Sauce)
Nacho Daddy
Knockemstiff, Ohio

Slaps you up just like Mom used to do.

Ingredients:
2 Cubano peppers
1 red bell pepper
1 jalapeno pepper
2 habanero peppers
1 serrano pepper
1 large yellow onion
1 can tomato paste (smoother style) or whole tomatoes and their juice (chunkier style)
Fresh cilantro
1/2 cup white vinegar
sun dried tomatoes
1/4 cup sugar
chipotle peppers with a little of their juice
3 cloves garlic

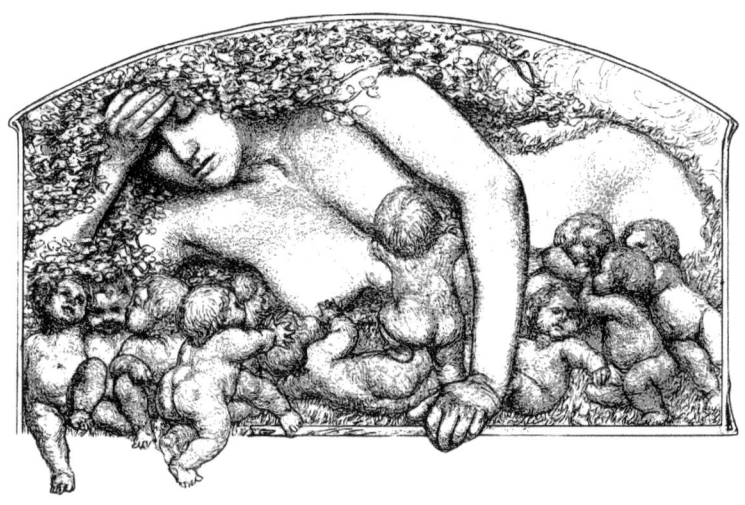

Instructions:
Roast the Cubanos, bell pepper, and onion until they get a nice charred flavor. Mince the garlic, remaining peppers, sun-dried tomatoes, chipotle peppers, and cilantro and throw everything into a big pot over medium high heat.

Let everything get nice and seared before stirring. When everything starts to soften and brown, add the tomato paste and season with sugar, cumin, turmeric, paprika, salt, and curry powder. Let simmer on medium heat about 15 minutes, covered. The longer it simmers the better.

Throw everything in the blender, in batches if necessary, and set aside.

Add the vinegar and strain until desired consistency is reached. Then add the cumin, turmeric, paprika, salt, and curry powder to taste.

Slap away until the cows come home, or you run out of slap sauce, or kids!

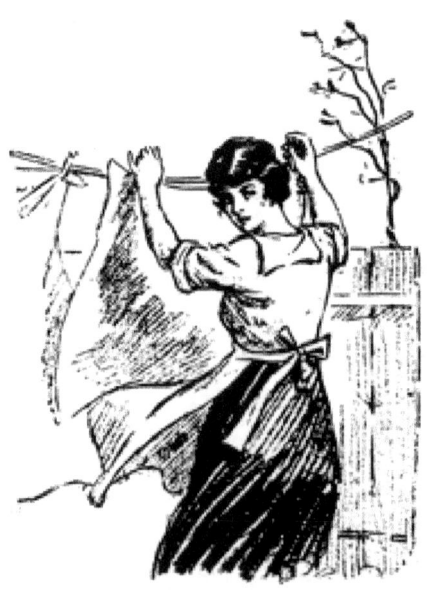

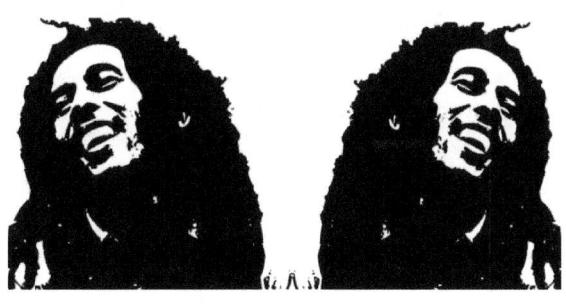

Marley's Smokin' Oh Juice
Jamaica Mi Krazy Kafe
Mexican Water, AZ.

Mexican Water is a piping hot, little town full of over-sunned locals. It's the only place in America that pumps Reggae music through little speakers hanging from poles all around town.

Town motto:
"Some say it's the water, others say it's the wine… still, others say …okay, we forgot what the others said, but it's a fun place to live."

Well, whatever it was, Marley's Smokey Oh Juice is definitely Jamaican Me Krazy!

Ingredients:
1- Lg. Onion,
4-5 Carrots,
3-4 Ribs Celery
3-4 Peeled Cloves of Garlic
2 tsp tomato paste,
½ tsp dry thyme (4-5 sprigs Fresh)
1-2 ea. bay leaf

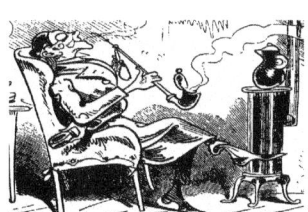

Instructions:
Clean and cut it all up, Mon. Din toss it all into da pan. Toss da beef, and let the ho ding smoke for one hour. Smoke up ya self, Mon while yer waiting for time to pass. Then get up, stand up" then …
Add 4-6 cups beef broth (to the beat my friends!)

Finish the Smoking process if yer eyez aren't too red by now, Mon!

While da roast is resting, dump da pan of da veggies juices and all into da pot and add 1 cup of da red wine, something you like to be drinkin' lots of, Mon.

Bring da *Oh Juice* to a boil din lower da heat and let it simma for 20-30 minutes. Strain out da veggies and let da *Oh Juice* rest a minute or so. All da fat will float to da top, Mon. Skim off da bulk of da fat. Ya can be using strips of da paper towels to drag quickly across to take off da last little bit of da fat.

Da purpose of smokin' da veggies a hour before addin' da broth and da herbs is cuz...the smoked out vegetables roasted in da supa dry heat concentrates da flavors and da sweetness giving da finished *Oh Juice* dat richer, deeper, fuller flava all da peeples luv.

Serve da sliced beef oh Juice or thicken the Jus to make da real cool gravy. Serve the sliced beef Oh Juice or thicken the Jus to make Gravy. Throw in a side of buttered to death veggies and ka-boom! Deliciousness in the desert! I say their motto should be:

"Since the accident I never thought I could look at meat again, but the Marley's Smokin' Oh Juice has given me hope! Don't miss out on slathering this stuff on a great big-O burgers and other gnarly meats! Mmmmmm!"
   -Terry "One ball" Stevenson - Ozark, MO.

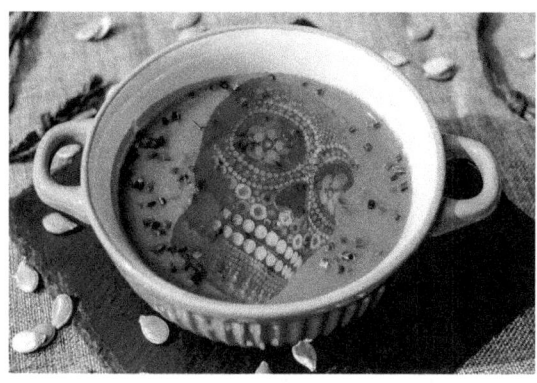

SOUP FOR THE DEAD
(CHICKEN TORTILLA SOUP)
NIN COM SOUP
CACA DEL TORO, MEXICO

A traditional *Dia de Muertos* or *Day of The Dead* dish (a fantastic Mexican holiday celebrating their dearly deceased.) You no longer have to be at the *Nin Com Soup* in Mexico to get it. Just run right out… or stumble like a zombie out and get.

Ingredients:
1 (46 ounce) can chicken broth
1 (15 ounce) can tomato sauce
1 (15 ounce) can diced tomatoes
3 cups cooked chicken, shredded (I use rotisserie from the deli)
2 Anaheim chilies, diced
1 jalapeno pepper, diced
1/2 cup diced onion
3-4 large tomatoes, diced
2 garlic cloves, minced
2 tablespoons minced cilantro
1 tablespoon chili powder
2 teaspoons cumin
2 teaspoons pepper
1 teaspoon salt
2 teaspoons Tabasco sauce (I use the chipotle flavor)
1/2 teaspoon chipotle pepper (optional)

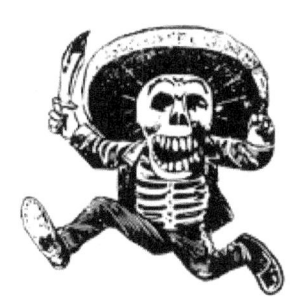

Garnish
1 cup shredded cheddar cheese
1 avocado, chopped
1/4 cup cilantro, pulled from stem
1 lime, cut into wedges
2 cups crushed tortilla chips

Instructions:
Throw everything except the garnishes into a Crockpot and let it cook on high for 5-6 hours.

Dress with garnishes and give it a squeeze of lime (a must:-)) and you're good to go!

If you are not using a crockpot, sauté the garlic and onion in 2 tablespoons olive oil before adding the remaining ingredients. Simmer for at least an hour so that the flavors mix really well.

The best part is now you can make it at home, and you won't have to share it with any "late relatives."

> *"Soup is just a way of screwing you out of a meal."*
> - Jay Leno

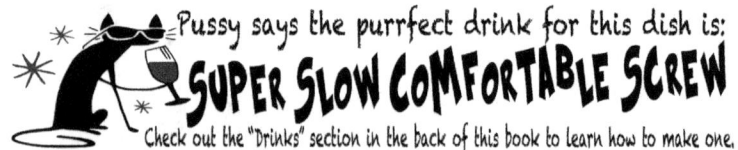
Pussy says the purrfect drink for this dish is: SUPER SLOW COMFORTABLE SCREW
Check out the "Drinks" section in the back of this book to learn how to make one.

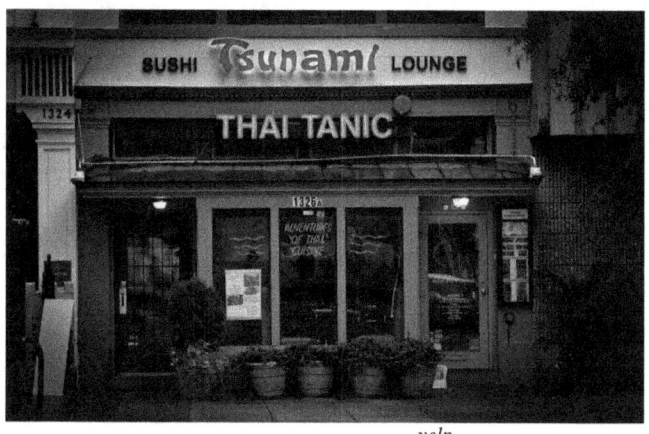
yelp

LEEKIE COCK SOUP
THAI TANIC RESTAURANT
TOLEDO, OHIO

Nobody likes a leaky cock. But out of all the leaky cock I've had in my mouth this is by far the best.

I can still feel it dribbling down my chin and staining my shirt.

Don't miss their *Three Legged Monkey* cocktail! I don't know what's in it. I just know my hair it's growing back!

Ingredients:
2 cups cooked chicken cubed (I used leftover rotisserie chicken)
3 leeks green top removed, sliced
1 large onion chopped
2 cloves garlic minced
2 ribs celery sliced
3 large potatoes peeled and cubed
2 large carrots peeled and sliced
48 oz. container chicken broth
fresh parsley to taste
Salt and pepper to taste
1 tsp. thyme
1 large bay leaf or two small bay leaves
fresh, snipped chives for garnish, if desired

fresh parsley for garnish, if desired

Instructions:
Place chicken, leeks, onion, garlic, celery, potatoes, carrots and chicken broth in a large crockpot. Add salt and pepper, parsley, thyme and a bay leaf.

Cook on low about 5 hours.

Remove to individual bowls and garnish with fresh parsley and snipped chives.

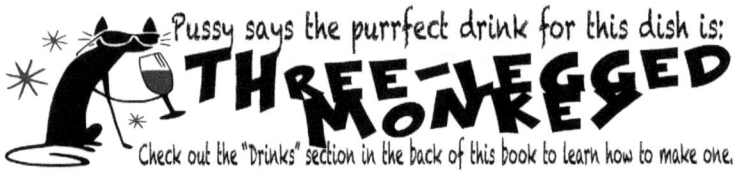
Pussy says the purrfect drink for this dish is: **THREE-LEGGED MONKEY**
Check out the "Drinks" section in the back of this book to learn how to make one.

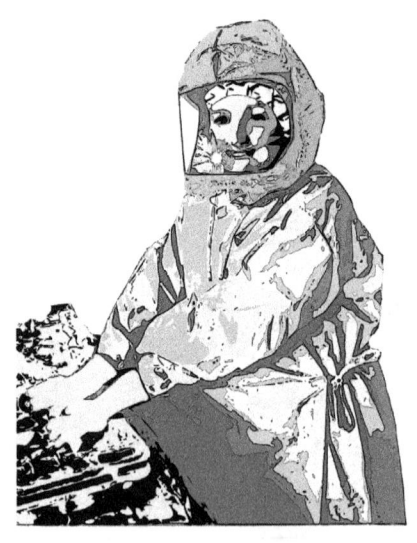

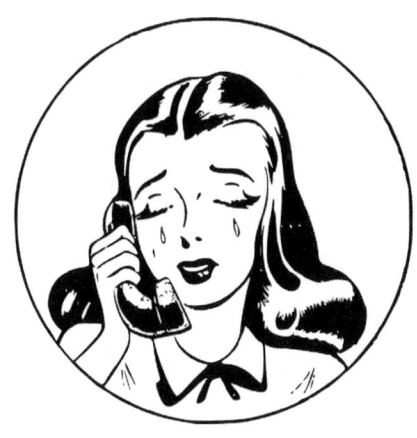

Happy Onions in Herbs Ball Sack
Town Cry Here Onion Bar
Sheep Boot, MA.

Here they specialize in onions. I mean all sorts of onions. They got purple onions, red onions, whites onions but what they're really famous for is their *Happy Onions in a Ball Sack!*

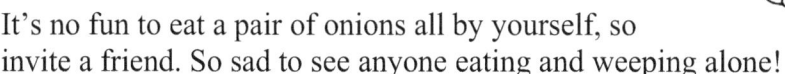

It's as fun as it sounds! A dish people come from miles around to cry over. A river of red wine and tying your onions up in cheesecloth makes this dish exceedingly exceptional.

It's no fun to eat a pair of onions all by yourself, so invite a friend. So sad to see anyone eating and weeping alone!

Ingredients:
For 18 to 24 peeled white onions about 1 inch in diameter:
1 1/2 tablespoons butter
1 1/2 tablespoons oil
A 9- to 10-inch enameled skillet
1/2 cup of brown stock, canned beef bouillon, dry white wine, red wine or water
Salt and pepper to taste
Don't forget a box of tear-wiping tissues.

Instructions:
Make a medium herb sack: 3 parsley springs, 1/2 bay leaf, and 1/4 teaspoon thyme tied in cheesecloth.

When the butter and oil are bubbling in the skillet, add the onion and sauté over moderate heat for about 10 minutes, rolling the onions about so they will brown as evenly as possible.

Be careful not to break their skins. You cannot expect to brown them uniformly. Pour in the liquid, season to taste, and add the herb bouquet.

Cover and simmer slowly for 40 to 50 minutes until the onions are perfectly tender but retain their shape, and the liquid has evaporated.

Remove the herb bouquet. Serve them as they are.

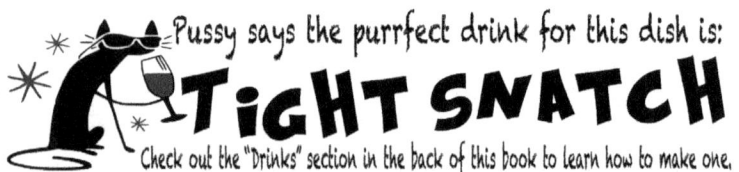

Pussy says the purrfect drink for this dish is: **TiGHT SNATCH**
Check out the "Drinks" section in the back of this book to learn how to make one.

"I have to admit I totally misread those instructions. Probably because I broke into the red wine a lil' early. My kids will tell you it was nine in the A.M. but I swear I was watchin' The Price is Right and everyone's knows that's on at ten! In any case, I just want to remind everyone to wrap up the <u>right onions</u> and tie up <u>the right sack!</u> Don't ask!"
   -Sam "Nine Toe" Smith

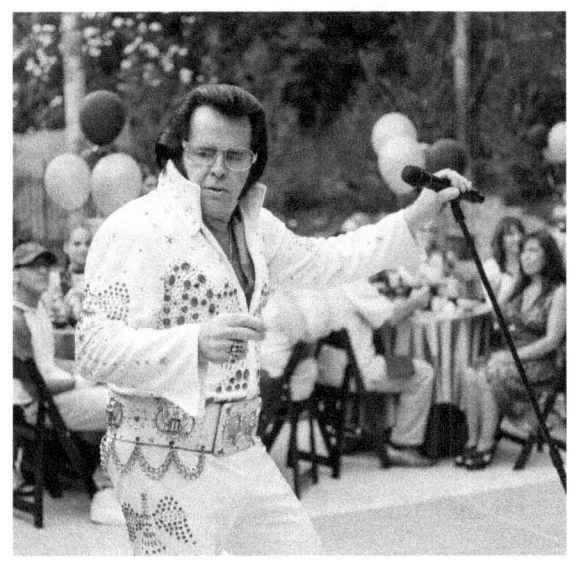

Sofa King Faking It

We get it! Some don't like to eat cock or other foul things. It is really amazing what some folks will put in their mouths! We agree. It's not for everyone. All of us here at *"How to Eat Cock The Sofa King Easy Way"* will stand by our motto, "Don't knock it, until you've tried it …at least twice! Just to be sure you did something wrong the first time"

But out of the goodness of our hearts (and pressure from the publisher) and to help you fit in, we've included for you this little section of recipes so you can really fake it! Go ahead, scream, and yell. No one is going to question it. Just go it!

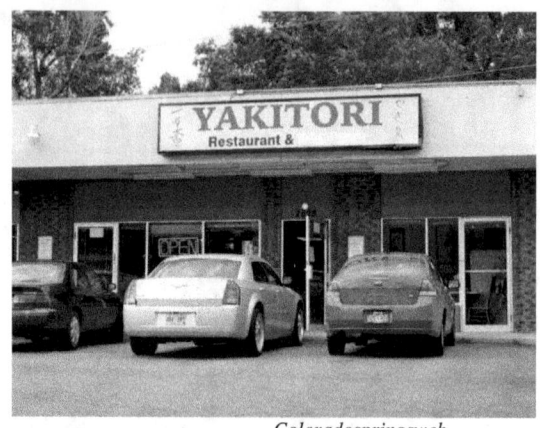
Coloradospringsweb

Worlds Best Yakitori Sauce & Chicken Skewers
Yakitori
Colorado Springs, Colorado
Andrea The Kitchen Witch

Here in Colorado Springs, there's an excellent little Japanese restaurant that I've been going to for over 25 years now called *The House of Yakitori*. They serve, yes that's right, Yakitori! Yakitori for those of you who don't know is skewered pieces of chicken, cooked over a charcoal grill, glazed with a delightful sweet sauce that is similar to teriyaki. Yakitori sauce is thicker, richer and a lot more flavorful than teriyaki sauce.

Instructions:
Yakitori sauce
makes about 8 servings
1/2 cup soy sauce
1/2 cup mirin
1/2 cup brown sugar
1/2 cup water
2 T rice vinegar
2 cloves garlic whole, crushed with back of knife

Combine everything in a sauce pan and bring to a boil. Reduce the heat and simmer.

Remove garlic cloves after 5 minutes of simmering.

Continue to cook until sauce has reduced and is a thick syrup.

CHICKEN SKEWERS:
1 lb chicken thighs boneless and skinless, cleaned and cut into chunks for skewering
2 T yakitori sauce
1 T soy sauce
bamboo skewers, soaked in water a minimum of 30 min before grilling

Marinate chicken in the sauces for 1 hour. While chicken marinates, soak the bamboo skewers in water. The moister the skewers are the fewer chances there is that they'll burn up on the grill.

Skewer about 2 oz of chicken on each skewer.

Grill over hot charcoal until done.
Drizzle with yakitori sauce when finished.

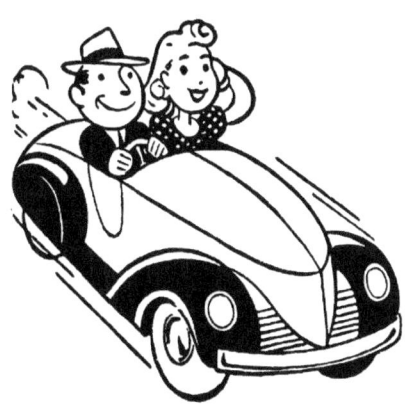

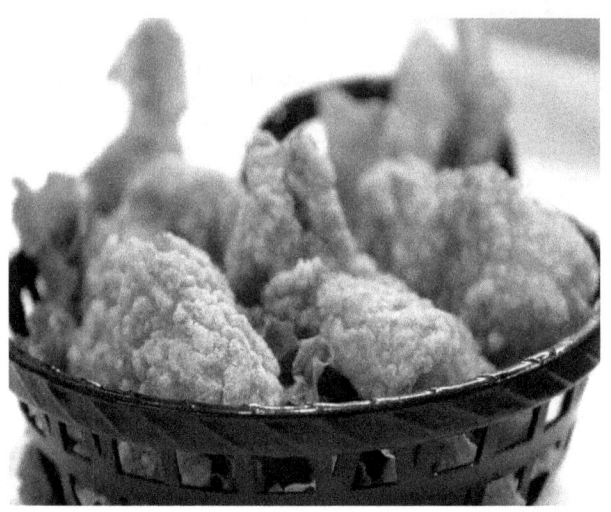

KFC's Original Fried Chicken

Ingredients:
1 large egg (beaten)
1 cup buttermilk
1 (3-pound) chicken (cut into 6 pieces)
1 cup all-purpose flour
1 teaspoon ground oregano
1 teaspoon chili powder
1 teaspoon dried sage
1 teaspoon dried basil
1 teaspoon dried marjoram
1 teaspoon pepper
2 teaspoons salt
2 tablespoons paprika
1 tablespoon onion salt
1 teaspoon garlic powder
2 tablespoons *Accent* ™ (MSG seasoning)
1 can lard, enough to cover chicken in the fryer

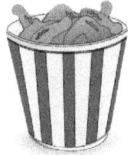

Instructions:
Combine the egg and buttermilk in a large bowl. Soak the chicken pieces in the mixture. Put the flour in a separate bowl and whisk in all the herbs and spices.

Remove the chicken from the buttermilk mixture, letting the excess drip off. Roll the chicken in the seasoned flour until completely covered.

Add the lard to a pressure fryer and heat to 365 F. Be sure to follow the manufacturer's directions.

Using a utensil, lower 4 pieces of the chicken into the hot oil and lock the lid in place. Be careful not to burn yourself with the hot oil.

Fry for 8 to 10 minutes, until the chicken is golden brown and thoroughly cooked. Once the pieces are cooked, release the pressure according to the manufacturer's directions and remove the chicken to paper towels or a metal rack to drain.

Repeat with the remaining 2 pieces of chicken.

Tips:
Although you may not be a fan of using MSG, the real secret to making this taste like the original Kentucky Fried recipe is including the *Accent* in the recipe, so do not eliminate this if you want authentic flavor. For even more authenticity, actually speak in the Colonel's deep Southern accent as you cook it up.

To assure the coating will stick, allow the chicken to sit for 20 to 30 minutes after rolling in the flour mixture.

Using a pressure fryer is key to creating the KFC crispiness; make sure the fryer temperature is at 365° before cooking the chicken.
To avoid making a mess and burning yourself, use a utensil when adding the chicken so's yer hands won't get Southern-fried!

Quickly lock the lid on the pressure fryer once all the pieces of chicken have been added.

If you can't get your hands on a pressure fryer, you can use a deep fryer; add enough vegetable oil or lard to keep the chicken pieces submerged and set the temperature to 350°.

Fry for 15 to 18 minutes, until golden brown and crispy. For crispier chicken use Crisco (one 3-pound can) instead of lard and double-coat the chicken with the flour mixture. That's the way the old Colonel liked it!

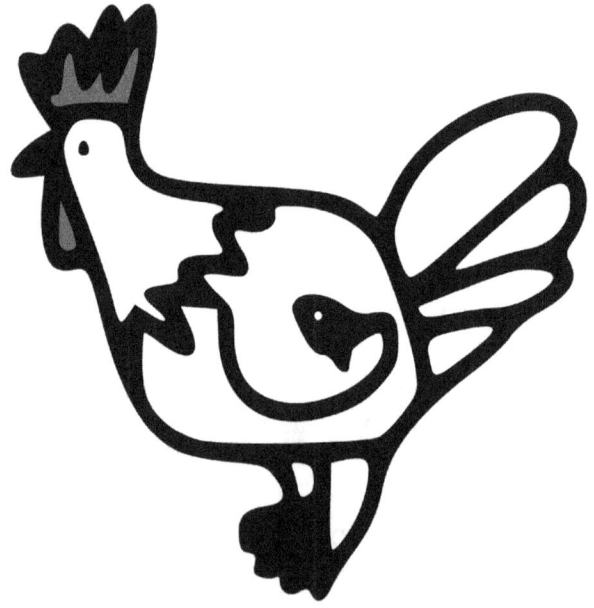

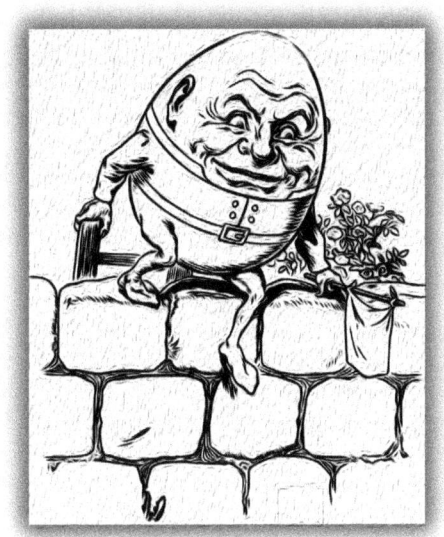

Star Bucks egg bites

The truffle aroma and fluffy texture make this a very tasty treat, especially if you add a few truffle shavings to the mixture.

Ingredients:
5 eggs (300 g total)
125 g ricotta cheese
125 g thick cream
50 g truffle parmesan cheese
½ tsp salt
1 tsp truffle oil
1 smoked pickled mushroom
1 slice semi-dried tomato
2–3 stalks garlic chives
6 small (4 oz) sterilized mason jars

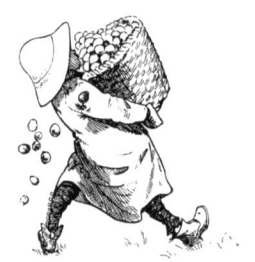

Instructions:
Grate cheese, and combine with cream, ricotta, eggs, and salt. Blend the mixture until perfectly smooth.

Slice mushroom and tomato into six pieces each and place one piece of each of into each jar. Fill jars with egg mixture. Drop three or four short pieces of garlic chives on top of the mixture for decoration. Add a few drops of truffle oil to each jar.

Loosely seal mason jars and cook at 75 °C for 40 minutes.
For a more intense truffle aroma, add a few shavings of black or white truffle to the mixture and keep it in a sealed container in the fridge for 24 hours before filling the jars.

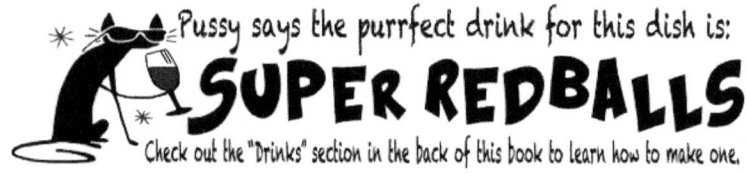

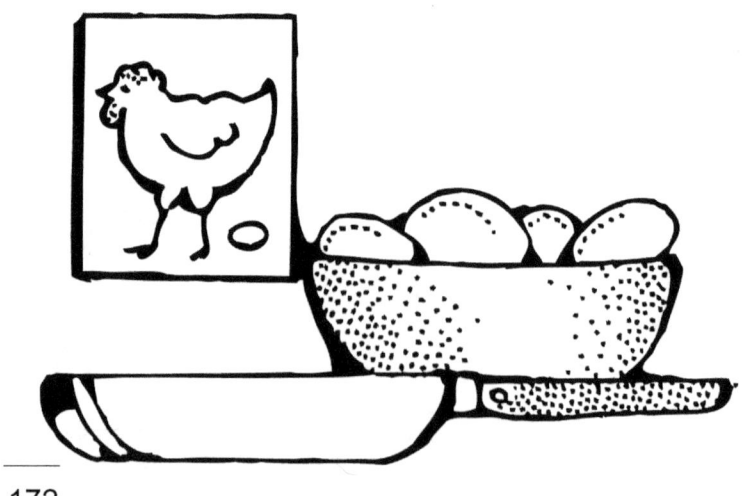

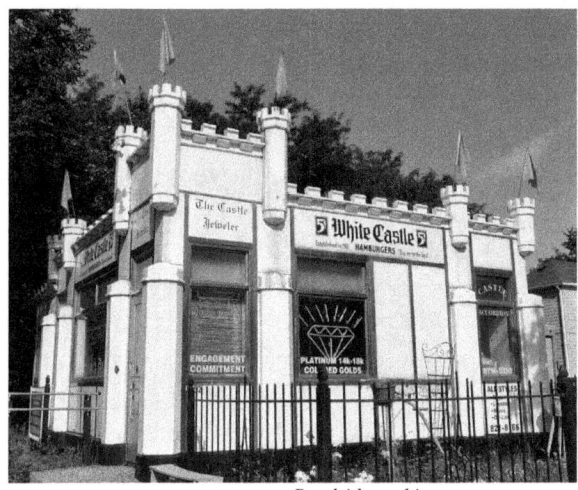
Roadside architecture

WHITE CASTLE SLIDERS

No better slider in the world! You must slide these into your mouth and often. These *White Castle* Sliders are friggin' delicious!

For those of you who have always wanted to duplicate these babies at home, this recipe is the real deal for 12 sliders.

Ingredients:
1 1/2 lbs. ground beef
1 envelope Lipton onion soup mix
1 tablespoon peanut butter (Yes, peanut butter. Trust me.
1/2 cup milk
1 onion finely chopped
1 dozen Sara Lee Classic Dinner Rolls or the really soft small-sized dinner rolls from the bakery, sliced in half
Cheese slices Kraft or Velveeta cheese slices work great.

Instructions:
In a large bowl mix the ground beef, Lipton onion soup mix, peanut butter, and milk. Spread the meat mixture on a cookie sheet. Use a rolling pin to roll over the meat to smooth it out.

Bake at 350 degrees for about 10 minutes. The meat will shrink. Take it out of the oven and put the diced onions all around the edges, this will give the meat a great flavor.

Bake for 15 more minutes, remove from oven, then spoon the onions from the edges all over the top of the meat and layer with cheese slices. Bake another 7-10 minutes (until cheese is melted).

Remove from oven and add the tops of the rolls (the bottom part of the rolls will just sit on the counter) and place back in the oven for about 5 more minutes.
Take it out of the oven. Slice the meat with a pizza cutter and pick up the slider/top bun with a spatula and set it on the bottom bun.

Serve immediately

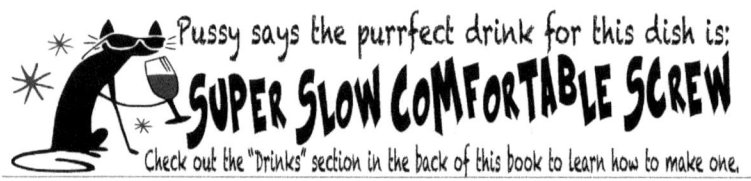

If you don't do anything stupid when you're young, you won't remember something funny when you're old...
   -Unknown

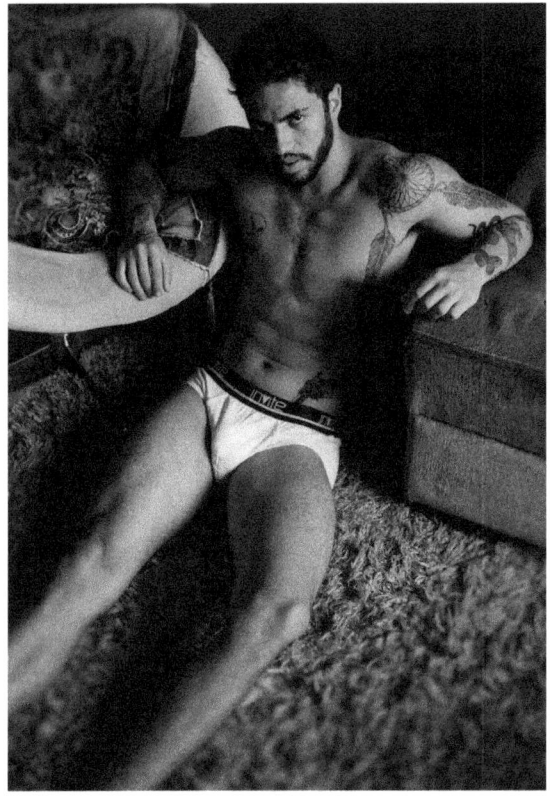

Steve's Sweet and Salty Hot Nuts

Sometimes I just get a craving for nuts. Not just any nuts but Steve's nuts. Whenever I get nut crazy I just whip up a batch of *Steve's sweet and salty hot nuts*.

Ingredients:
2 1/4 cups (18-ounces) assorted unsalted nuts like peanuts, cashews, Brazil nuts, hazelnuts, walnuts, pecans, whole almonds or just about any nuts you enjoy putting in your mouth.
2 tablespoons coarsely chopped fresh rosemary leaves
1/2 teaspoon cayenne pepper
2 teaspoons dark brown sugar
2 teaspoons sea salt
1 tablespoon unsalted butter, melted

Instructions:
Preheat the oven to 350°.

Toss your nuts in a large bowl to combine and spread them out on a baking sheet. Toast in the oven until light golden brown, about 10 minutes.

In a large bowl, combine the rosemary, cayenne, sugar, salt, and melted butter. Thoroughly toss the toasted nuts in the spiced butter and serve warm. And once you eat these, you will never want to stop.

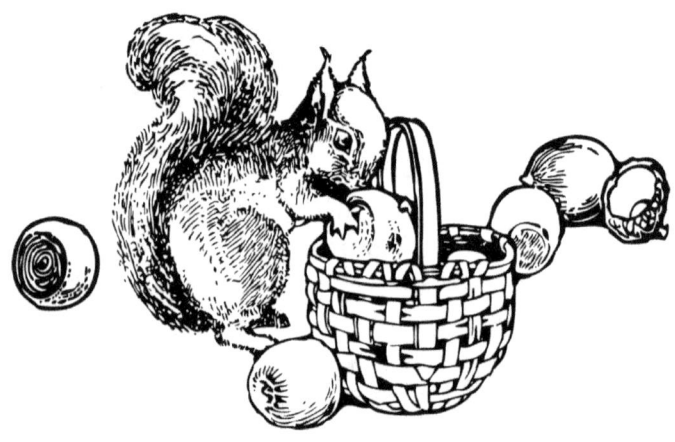

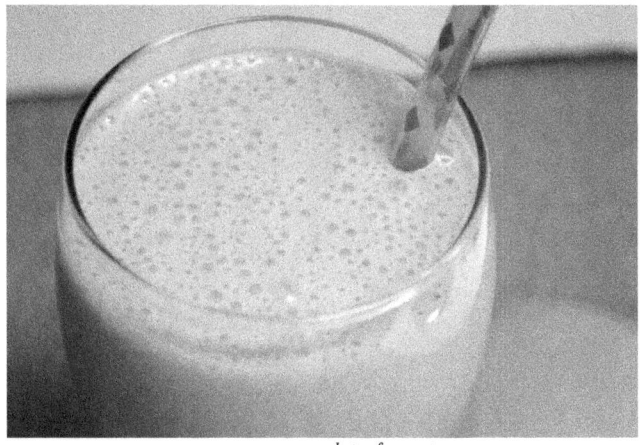
glutenfreecat.com

ORANGE JULIUS

We've been making this *Orange Julius* copycat drink since we were kids. For an added twist, try adding fresh strawberries, raspberries, and or pineapple!

Ingredients:
1 can 6oz frozen orange juice concentrate
1 c. milk
1 c. water
1/4 c. sugar
2-3 Tbsp. powdered sugar
1 tsp vanilla
about 10-11 ice cubes

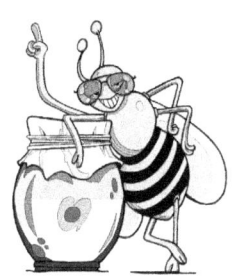

Instructions:
In a blender, blend all ingredients except ice. Slowly add ice cubes one at a time until it reaches a "smoothie" consistency. Serve immediately.

If you are adding frozen fruit, add a little at a time BEFORE adding ice cubes. If using fresh fruit, add at the very beginning when you are blending everything else.

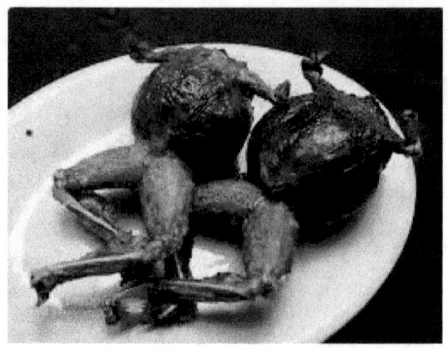

Quora
SIDE KICKS!
A side dish is a food item that accompanies the entrée or main course at a meal. Much like what Charlie Sheen is to Macaulay Culkin, what the Joker is to Carrot Top, or what Charles Manson is to Marilyn Manson.

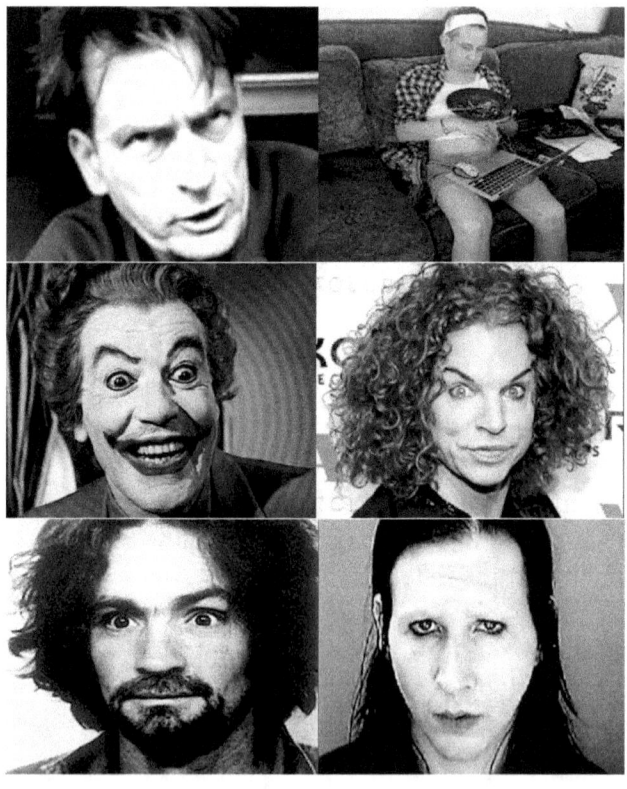

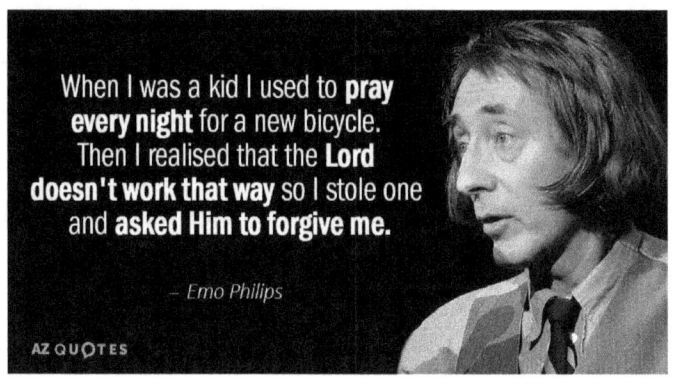

Emo Philip's Coleslaw Recipe
By Emo Philips

Instructions:
1. Chop cabbage into a large bowl.
2. Look for green peppers.
3. Drive to store.
4. Choose green peppers.
5. Carry them to the cashier.
6. Drive home.
7. Find wallet.
8. Drive to store.
9. Buy green peppers.
10. Drive home.
11. Chop green peppers into a bowl.
12. Look for mayonnaise.
13. Drive to store.
14. Buy mayonnaise.
15. Drive home.
16. Mix mayonnaise into a bowl.
17. Look for raisins.
18. Drive to store.
19. Buy stupid raisins.
20. Ignore stupid cashier's snickering.
21. Drive home.
22. Mix raisins into bowl.
23. Look for miserable lousy stupid carrots.

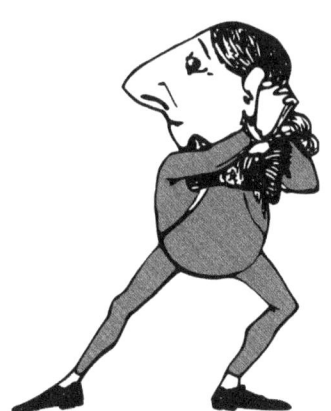

24. Drive to stupid lousy store.
25. Buy miserable stupid lousy carrots.
26. Call stupid miserable snickering cashier a Nazi.
27. Crawl to car.
28. Drive home.
29. Chop stupid damned miserable lousy carrots into a damned stupid lousy miserable bowl.
30. Look for finger.
31. Look harder for finger.
32. Look everywhere for finger.
33. See cat scurrying away.
34. Follow cat into new neighbor's house, surprising him in the middle of drug deal.
35. Dive over sofa to escape gunfire, landing on cat's tail, causing cat to screech and jump up into new neighbor's face and claw his eyes as he's bending over the sofa about to shoot you, enabling you to grab the gun from his hand, enabling you to hold the gun on him until the cops arrive, who then arrest him and drive you and the cat to the hospital where the cat's stomach is pumped, and your finger is found and sewn back on good as new.
36. Collect the reward of half of the neighbor's property from drug auction, then just buy all the delicious coleslaw you want from a nice deli.

You could and should find Emo here:
http://www.emophilips.com

"This whole thing 'bout scared me to death! I was having scary coleslaw dreams so I ran to my neighbor's and he calmed me down and made me a drink. One thing led to another and needless to say we got married and are expecting lil' Emo "Coleslaw"Ballrestchin and day now! Thanks Sofa King Easy!"
-*Cindy Ballrestchin of Malibu, CA.*

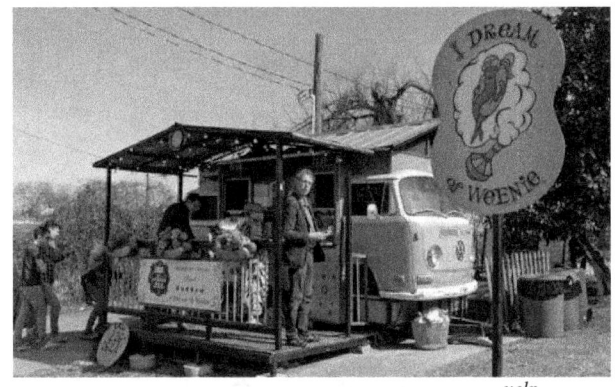
yelp

DIRTY TATER BITES
I DREAM OF WEENIE
BAKED, ALASKA

It's friggin' dark here most of the year. It's also too cold to take a shower. This very well could be the reason Eskimos came up with that whole just touching-noses thing!

Ingredients:
4 large baking potatoes
1 bag dry onion soup mix
Olive oil

Instructions:
Preheat oven to 400 degrees. And line a baking sheet with aluminum foil? Spray with non-stick cooking spray. Cut potatoes into bite-size pieces. Place in a bowl and sprinkle them with onion soup mix. Stir to coat.

Place in a single layer on a baking sheet. Drizzle with olive oil. Bake for 20-30 minutes or until forkin' tender. Use extra potatoes as pocket-warmers to help you make it to your car before freezing to death.

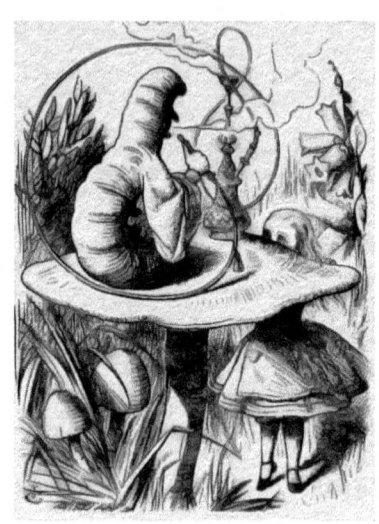

GREAT HEAD JOB
(SAUTÉED MUSHROOMS)
THE GOLDEN SPOON CAFÉ
DARNKIDS, FLORIDA

You can find killer shrooms just about anywhere, but no one does them up like these guys. Of course, the big fun comes in hunting the little guys.

This means a trip to a nearby jungle. Be ready for "Get outta the jeep." "Get back in the jeep!" "Watch out for that snake!" "Do you know mouth-to-mouth?!" and "Can you land a helicopter?!"

Ten hours later we arrive back at *The Golden Spoon Café* to slather ourselves up in calamine lotion and the mushrooms up in butter! So worth it!

Ingredients:
1/2 pound fresh mushrooms
2 tablespoons butter
1 tablespoon oil
1 to 2 tablespoons minced shallots or green onions (optional)
Salt and pepper

Instructions:
Place a skillet over high heat with the butter and oil.

As soon as you see the butter foam has begun to subside, indicating that it is hot enough, add the mushrooms. (Leave whole if small, sliced or quartered if large.) Toss and shake the pan for 4 to 5 minutes. During their sauté the mushrooms will at first absorb the fat.

In 2 to 3 minutes, the fat will reappear on their surface, and the mushrooms will begin to brown. As soon as they have browned lightly, remove from heat. Let cool and serve.

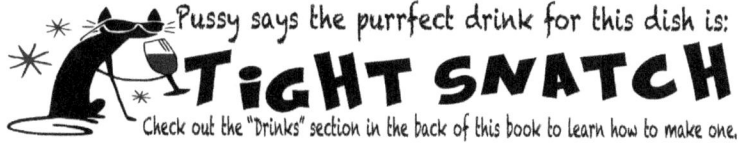
Pussy says the purrfect drink for this dish is: **TIGHT SNATCH**
Check out the "Drinks" section in the back of this book to learn how to make one.

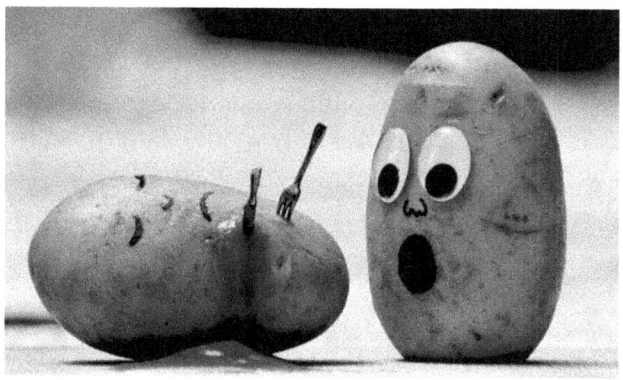

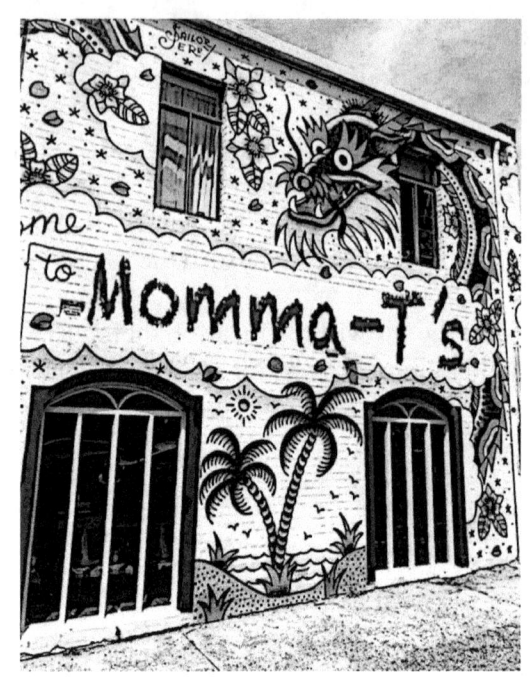

Momma-T's Tater Tot Casserole
Momma-T's
Bumpass, VA.

Momma-T's has more on their menu than mouth-watering cock and desserts most can only dream about, they also have *Momma-T's Tater Tot Casserole*. Kids go nuts for this stuff. Go ahead order up but don't expect to finish up. One order of piping hot *MTTTC* could feed a family of four!

FUN FACT:
The name *Momma-T's* was supposed to be "*Manatees*" (the animal). Turns out Rey-Rey (the painter) was not only a little hard of hearing but a bit of a drinker as well.

Ingredients:
1 1/2 pounds ground beef
1 (16-ounce) package frozen tater tot
1 tablespoon olive oil
1 onion, diced
1 (15-ounce) can black beans, drained and rinsed
1 cup corn kernels, frozen, canned or roasted
1 cup salsa, homemade or store-bought
1 (4.5-ounce) can chopped green chilies drained
1 tablespoon taco seasoning mix
1 (10-ounce) can mild enchilada sauce
3/4 cup shredded sharp cheddar cheese
2 tablespoons chopped fresh cilantro leaves

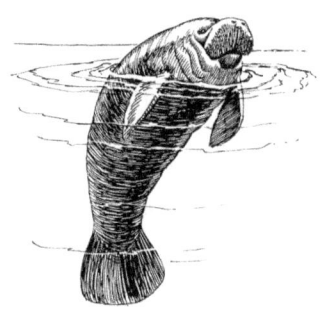

Instructions:
Heat olive oil in a large skillet over medium high heat.

Add ground beef and onion and cook until beef has browned, about 3-5 minutes, making sure to crumble the beef as it cooks; drain excess fat and remove from heat.

Stir in black beans, corn, salsa, green chilies, taco seasoning and enchilada sauce. Lightly coat the inside of a 4-qt slow cooker with nonstick spray. Spread half of your taters onto the bottom of the slow cooker; top with ground beef mixture and remaining tater tots.

Cover and cook on low heat for 3-4 hours. Add cheese during the last 30 minutes of cooking time.

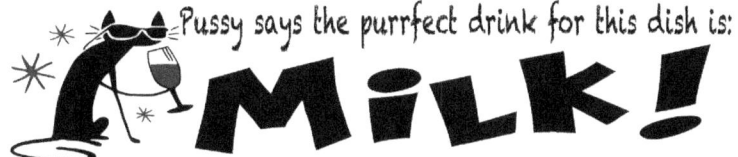

"I eat Momma T's everything, you know? She is a nice lady who never talks too loud and is always playing with her hot box. Good, yummy things come outta there every day, you know? And it's always hot, steamy and sticky but that's the way I like it, you know?"

-Rey-Rey (age 77) of Bumpass, VA.

MOMMA-T'S TATER TOT CASSEROLE IS WINNER OF: MOTHER'S DOING IT UP RIGHT AWARD!

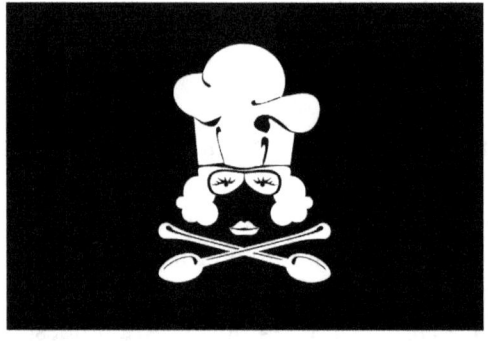

Congrats Momma!

"Momma Tat tators! Daaaaa!!!! Tata tata ta!"
-Lil' Jimmy Wiggins (age 3)

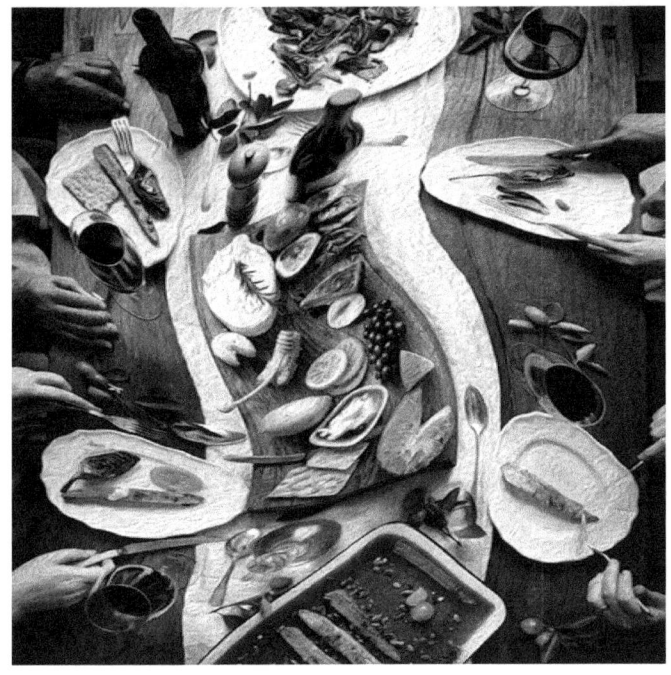

Appetizers (first bites)

You've finally made the decision to eat a big cock. Great! That first stroke is so important if you want to impress. It has to be something to get the salivary glands really pumping!

Here are some fun things you can put into your mouth to help get you in the mood.

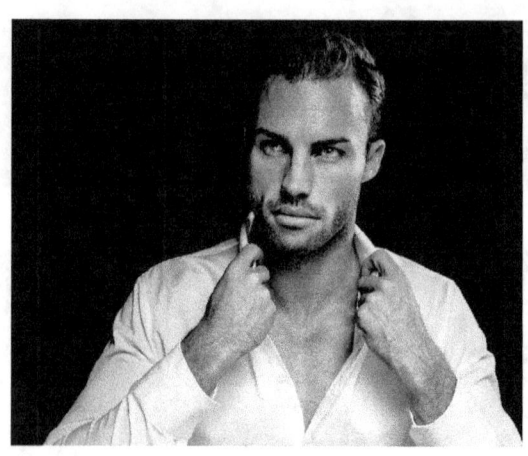

Pass Around My Sweet, Salty & Spicy Nuts
Wild Thyme Café Bar
Smithville, TN

There is nothing a man loves more then to have his *Sweet Salty Spicy Nuts* passed around a bar and popped into many hot awaiting mouths.

Ingredients:
Cooking spray
1 cup untoasted walnut halves
1 cup untoasted pecan halves
1 cup unsalted, dry roasted almonds
1 cup unsalted, dry roasted cashews
1 teaspoon salt
1/2 teaspoon freshly ground black pepper
1/4 teaspoon ground cumin
1/4 teaspoon cayenne pepper
1/2 cup white sugar
1/4 cup water
1 tablespoon butter

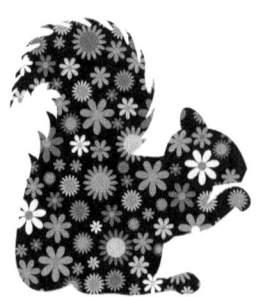

Instructions:
Preheat oven to 350°.

Line a baking tray with aluminum foil and coat it with cooking spray. Place your walnuts into a baggie. Add salt, black pepper, cumin, and cayenne pepper to your walnut sack with your other nuts. Toss and play with your nut sack until you feel like you have to stop.

Cook sugar, water, and melted butter over medium heat for 1 minute and remove from heat. Slowly pour butter mixture over your nuts and shake to coat. Transfer your slippery nuts to the prepared baking sheet and spread into a single layer.

Bake your nuts in the 350° oven for 10 minutes. Stir your nuts until the warm syrup coats every nut. Return to the oven, and bake until your nuts are sticky and roasted about 6 minutes.

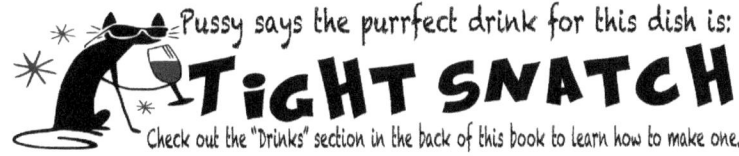

Pussy says the purrfect drink for this dish is: **TiGHT SNATCH**
Check out the "Drinks" section in the back of this book to learn how to make one.

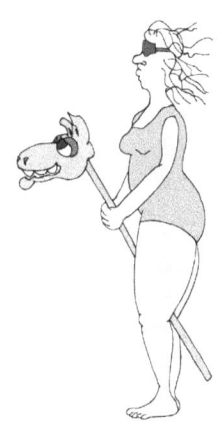

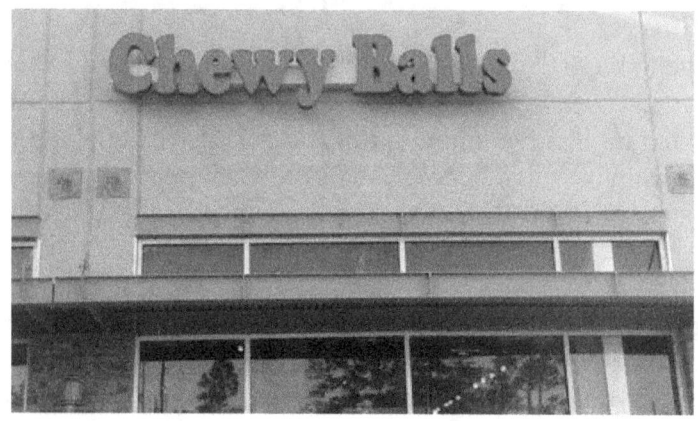

Chef's Chocolate Salty Balls
Chewy Balls
South Park, CO

Chef's Chocolate, Salty, Balls are world famous and they can be ball deep in your mouth too!

Ingredients:
2/3 cup salted butter
1 1/2 cups sugar
1/4 cup brandy
4 cups semisweet chocolate chips
2 teaspoons vanilla extract
4 eggs
2 tablespoons cinnamon
1 1/2 cups flour
1/2 teaspoon baking soda
1/2 teaspoon table salt
Kosher salt, to taste

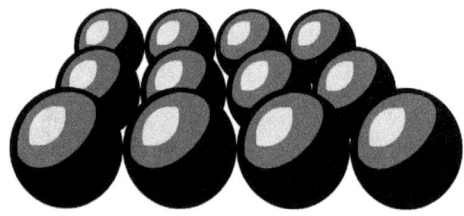

Instructions:
In a saucepan, bring the butter, sugar, and brandy to a boil, stirring constantly. Remove from the heat.
Stir (with a wooden spoon) in 2 cups of chocolate chips until melted and then take off the heat and stir in the vanilla.

In a large mixing bowl, beat the eggs. Gradually add the chocolate mixture and mix well.

In a separate bowl, combine the flour, baking soda, cinnamon, and salt, and then gradually add to the chocolate mixture.

Spread onto a greased baking pan and bake at 325 degrees for 35-45 minutes or until a fork inserted in the center comes out clean. Since your balls are black, it is easy to burn them.

On a plate spread out some kosher or sea salt. With a spoon scrape up a balls worth of mix depending if you like large or small balls. Rub your balls between your palms until satisfied. Then roll your balls into the sea salt. Remember a little salt on your balls goes a long way.

Invite your friends over to play with, suck on, and eat your balls. It makes for an entertaining evening no one will forget.

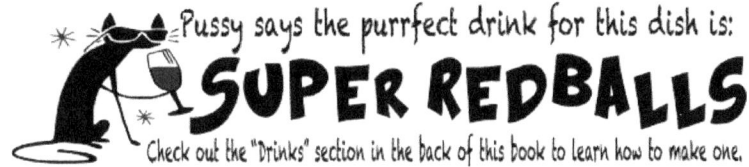

Pussy says the purrfect drink for this dish is: SUPER REDBALLS
Check out the "Drinks" section in the back of this book to learn how to make one.

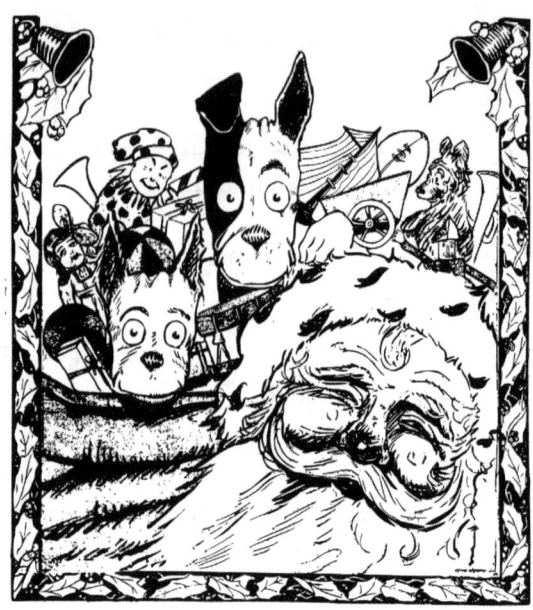

ST. CHRISTMAS CRACK NUTS
UNDER SANTA'S NORTH POLE

While it is not at the tip of Santa's North Pole, they are right down under it.

Nothing better than some suckable nuts on a cold winters night right? It is like crack for Mr. Peanut. A fully dressed cock surrounded by a cornucopia of tantalizing treats sure to set mouths a waterin'. I'd always heard that mint, crushed berries, maple syrup, and even brown sugar can significantly improve the taste of any cock big or small.

Ingredients:
2 jars unsalted or unsalted peanuts, 16 oz
1 bag semi-sweet chocolate chips, 12 oz
1 bag milk chocolate chips, 12 oz
2 bag peanut butter chips, 10 oz each
2 pkg white almond or vanilla candy coating, 1 lb each

Instructions:
Starting with your nuts layer, all the ingredients in a large Crock Pot putting the sweets on top. Cover with a lid and cook on low stirring every few minutes. Once the mixture looks like something, Rudolph left behind scoop it out with a spoon and leave the Christmas Crack nuts to harden before eating.

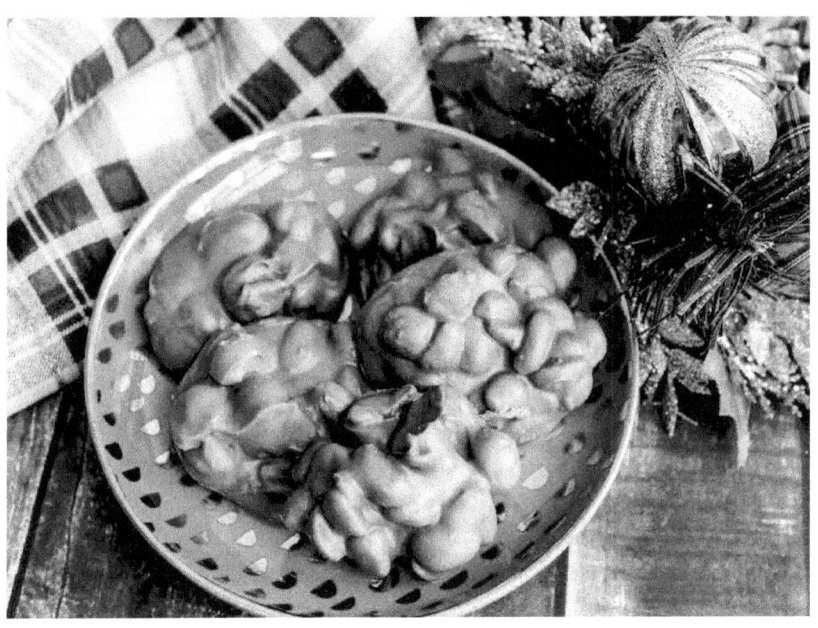

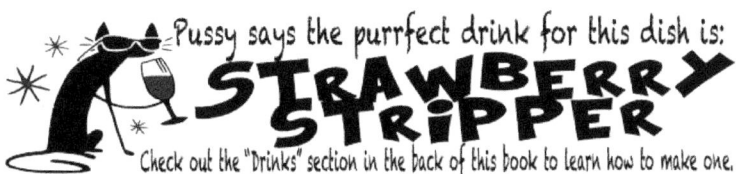

Pussy says the purrfect drink for this dish is: **STRAWBERRY STRIPPER**
Check out the "Drinks" section in the back of this book to learn how to make one.

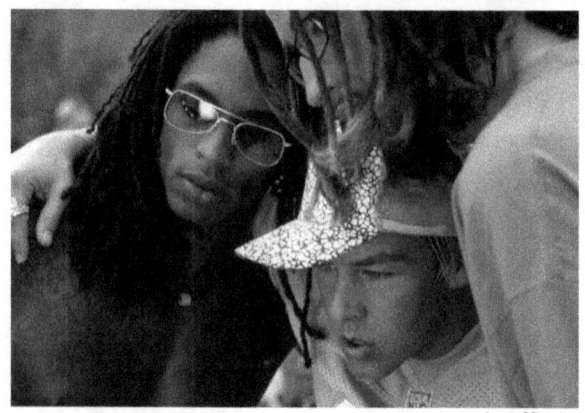
Angelfire

Swollen Members' Chocolate Walnut Shrimp
Turnip the Beet Café
Port Angeles, WA.

This place has it all! TV dinner trays sitting on Persian rugs Throw pillows, cubby-holes, and waitresses who can read lips. I don't want to say the sitar music is loud but. ….What?!!! You have no choice but to throw down on the *Swollen Members' Chocolate Walnut Shrimp*. It's so killer! It'll make you just want to turn it up, whip it out and crank it until you scream! Here's is the secret to making their signature dish!

Ingredients:
Shrimps - 8 tiger shrimps
3 cloves minced garlic,
1 small minced chili pepper
2 tablespoons walnut oil
1 orange juice
1/2 orange zest
Lemon juice - to taste (if orange is too sweet)
15 g Dark chocolate
3 tablespoons white wine -

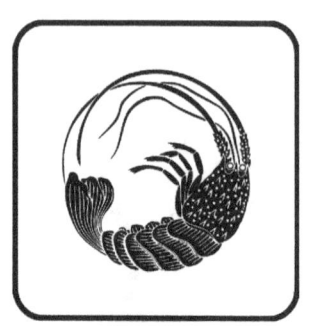

Instructions:

In a small pot, heat the orange juice, orange zest and wine. Do not boil! Immediately drink any leftover wine. "Wine not wasted ...Waste wine not.."

When it's hot, add the chocolate and remove from heat. Whisk the mixture to melt the chocolate. Add some lemon juice if the sauce is too sweet.

In a skillet, heat the oil and add garlic and chili.

Sauté for a minute, remove garlic and chili from oil, save the garlic mixture.

In the same skillet, add the shrimp to oil and sauté till the shrimp is done.

Pour the chocolate sauce into the skillet over the shrimp; add garlic and chili, sauté until the sauce thickens a little bit. Serve immediately. Stick that Choco-shrimp in your mouth and live the dream.

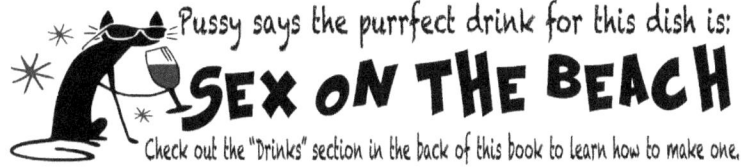

Pussy says the purrfect drink for this dish is: **SEX ON THE BEACH**
Check out the "Drinks" section in the back of this book to learn how to make one.

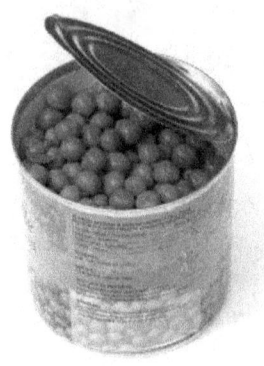

Canned Peas
King Soopers
No Name, Colorado

This is by far is the easiest recipe to cook in all of this book.

It may sound silly, but this one takes me back to my childhood where peas were not only a food but also a source of ammo. Wet green spoon-flipped projectiles flew across our dining room table right for my little brother's head. Good times.

Ingredients:
1 can of peas

Instructions:
1. Take can off of shelf.
2. Take can opener out of drawer.
3. Open can.
4. Set burner to high
5. Put pan on burner.
6. Add peas.
7. Cook until done.
8. Eat.

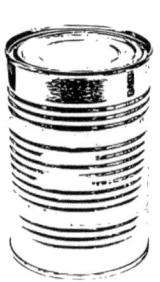

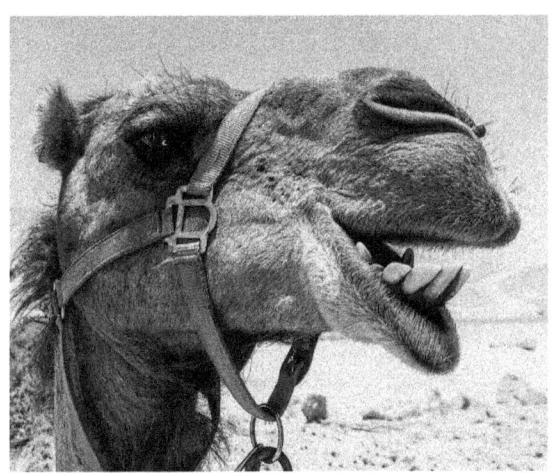

STUFF THAT CAMEL
SYRIAN DIPITY
DUSTMASKUS, SYRIA

How many times have you heard, "Hey! Go stuff that Camel!" Okay, I'd never heard it either, but I guess it's a term of endearment in some parts of the world.

Stuff, My Camel, is a really straightforward recipe and it'll feed a ton of people. Literally a ton! So pitch a tent. It may be "midnight at the oasis" but don't "send your camel to bed," we're gonna Stuff That Camel with a bunch of hot cocks!!!

Ingredients:
1 Medium Camel (You may need to special order this.)
4 Lambs (Check with the camel guy)
20 Roasted cocks
150 Boiled Eggs
40 Pounds of Tomatoes
Salt and Seasonings

Instructions:
1. Stuff eggs into tomatoes.
2. Stuff tomatoes into chickens.
3. Stuff chickens into lambs.
4. Stuff lambs into camel.
5. Roast until tender
6. Serve with a side of hummus and half a ton of hot pita bread.

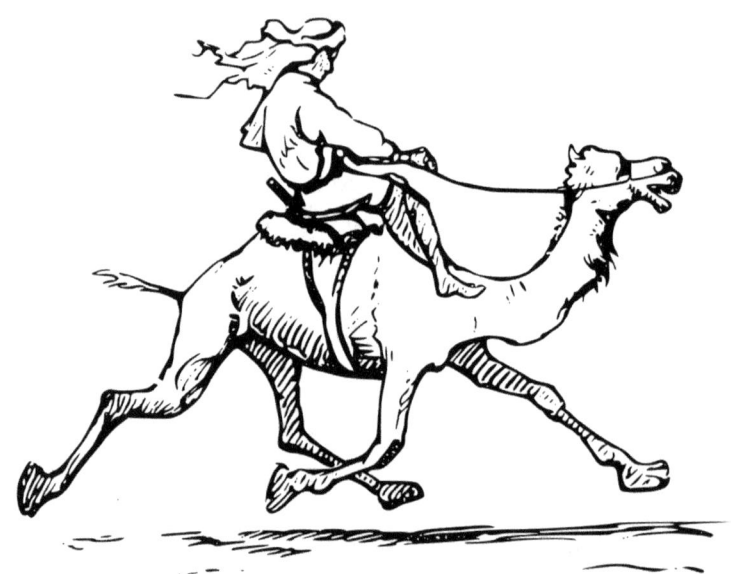

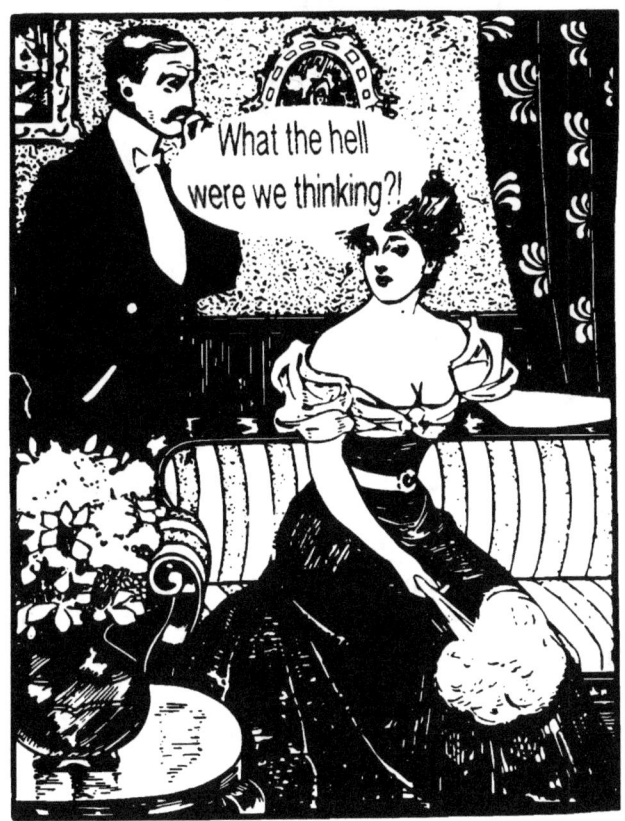

TOTALLY GROSS THINGS YOUR GRANDPARENTS PUT IN THEIR MOUTHS

What were they thinking? Back in the day, they'd eat stuff that would really freak people out today. Some of what you'll see here might seem strange, but there was a time people just couldn't wait to get this stuff into their mouths. Not highly recommended unless you're out to fool your friends but good.

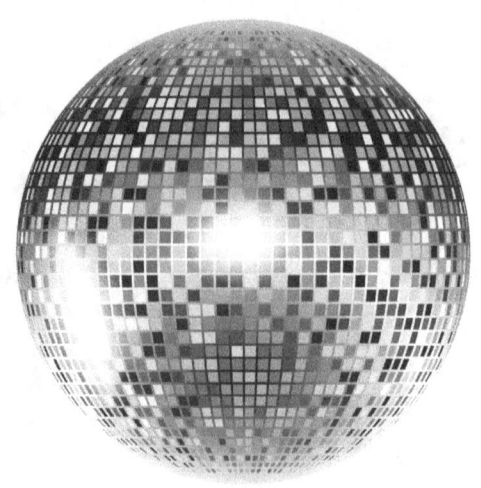

70s Diet Jellied Tomato Refresher

One of the many diet crazes from the '70s. Others included Onions and Lime Zest, Pea juice (you don't want to get that one wrong!) Wine Coolers with chunks of peaches or Rose Water and Vodka.

It was the height of the Disco, people would do just about anything to look good. My grandmother lost twenty pounds drinking this stuff. I heard she was adding more and more vodka to her "Rose Water" daily.

It all makes sense now. The fond memories of ole' granny smelling like Russian catsup.

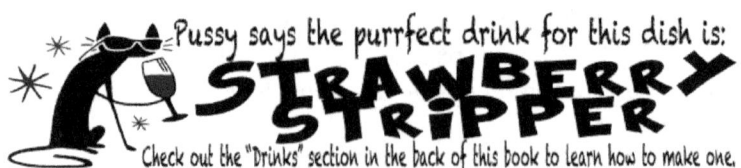

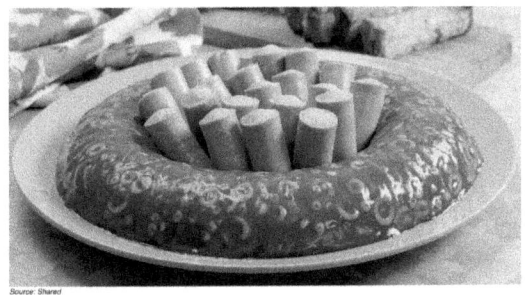
Source: Shared

UPRIGHT ORGAN PARTY

A real "party-stopper" in the mid 1950's. This is a giant *Jell-O* ring filled with childhood favorite *Spaghetti-Os*! The flavor is exactly as you remember, only it's cold like death instead of mouth-burning hot.

Serve it with some Vienna sausages upright in the ring! Try not to cringe when someone stabs one on the end with a toothpick. The hit of any gathering when people take turns trying to eat your sausages without using their hands!

Wow! Our grandparents lived on the edge!

Ingredients:
 ¼ cup water
 ¼ cup condensed tomato soup
 2 (¼ ounce) packets unflavored gelatin
 2 cans *Spaghetti-Os*

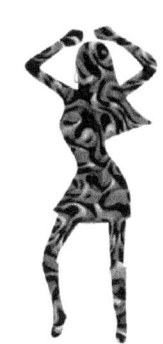

Instructions:
In a large pot, pour in your water and condensed tomato soup, then sprinkle the gelatin on top. Allow gelatin to bloom in the water, about 5-10 minutes.

Once the gelatin has bloomed, stir together lightly.
Place the pot on the stove and turn the heat to medium, then keep occasionally stirring until the gelatin has completely dissolved, and the mixture is quite smooth.

Turn off the heat and add the Spaghetti-Os to the pot. Mix until well-combined, then pour evenly into 4 cup ring mold.

Release from mold and add lil' wieners.

Laugh as you watch your friends munch it all down. Great food is like great sex. The more you have the more you want.
   - **Gael Greene**

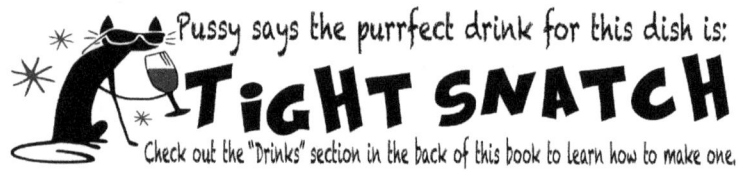

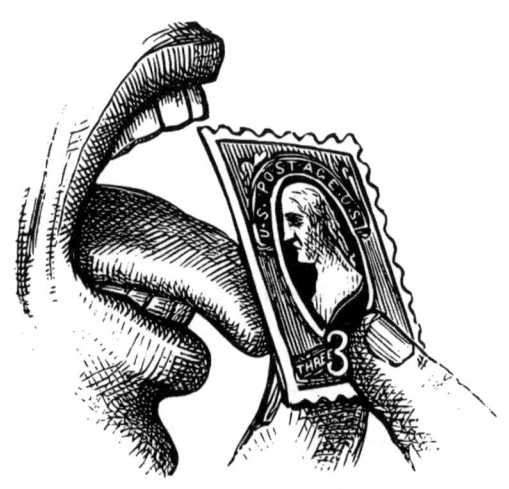

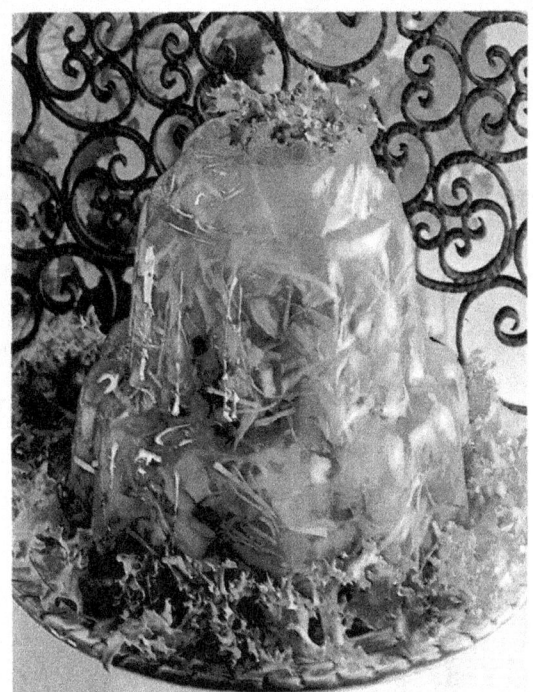

McCall's Great American Recipe Card Collection

Yawning in Technicolor
Veggie Fruit Salad

Maybe it's a "Surprise! A Jell-O mold filled with food remnants that are always found in the sink drain screens after a party. It was made famous in the great depression, and they were happy to have it.

Ingredients:
2 envelopes unflavored gelatin
1/2 cup sugar
1 teaspoon salt
'1 can (12 oz) apple juice
1/2 cup lemon juice
2 tablespoons vinegar
1 cup shredded carrot
1 cup sliced celery

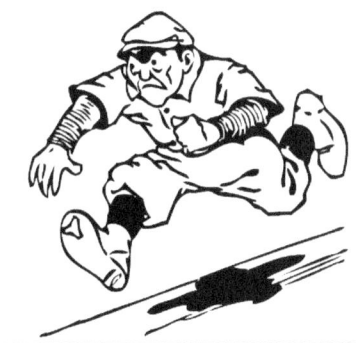

1 cup finely shredded cabbage
1/2 cup chopped green pepper
1 can (4 oz) chopped pimiento

Instructions:
In a small saucepan, combine gelatin, sugar, and salt; mix well.

Add 1 cup water. Heat over low heat, constantly stirring, until sugar and gelatin are dissolved. Remove from heat and stir in apple juice, lemon juice, vinegar, and 1/4 cup cold water. Pour into a medium bowl.

Refrigerate 1 hour, or until mixture is the consistency of unbeaten egg white.
Add carrot, celery, cabbage, green pepper, and pimiento; stir until well combined.

Turn into decorative, 1 1/2-quart mold. Refrigerate 4 hours, or until firm.

To unmold: Run a small spatula around edge of mold; invert onto a serving plate. Place hot dishcloth over mold; shake gently to release.

Repeat, if necessary. Liftoff the mold and refrigerate until ready to serve.

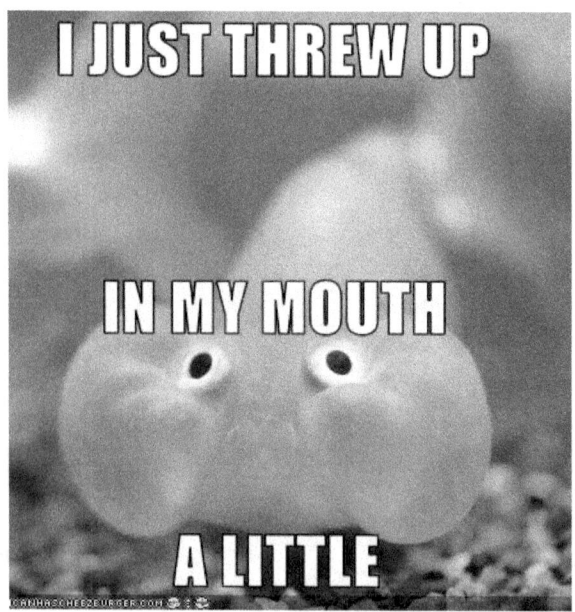

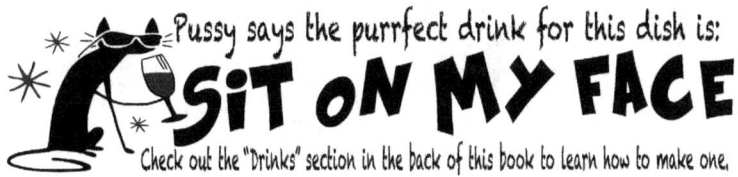

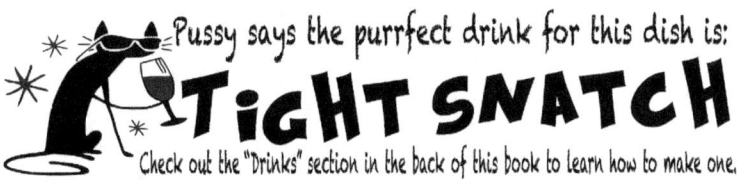

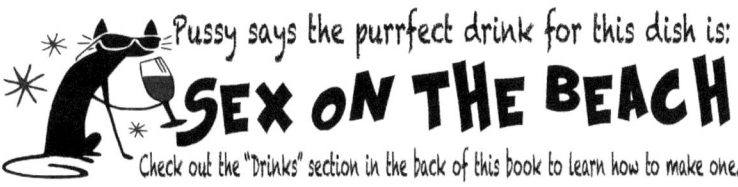

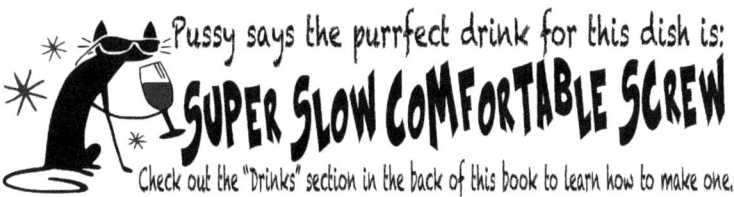

Yep! Drink all of these!

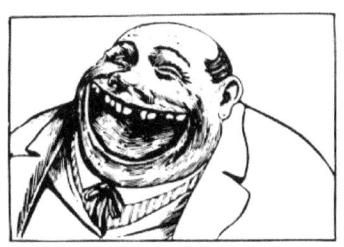

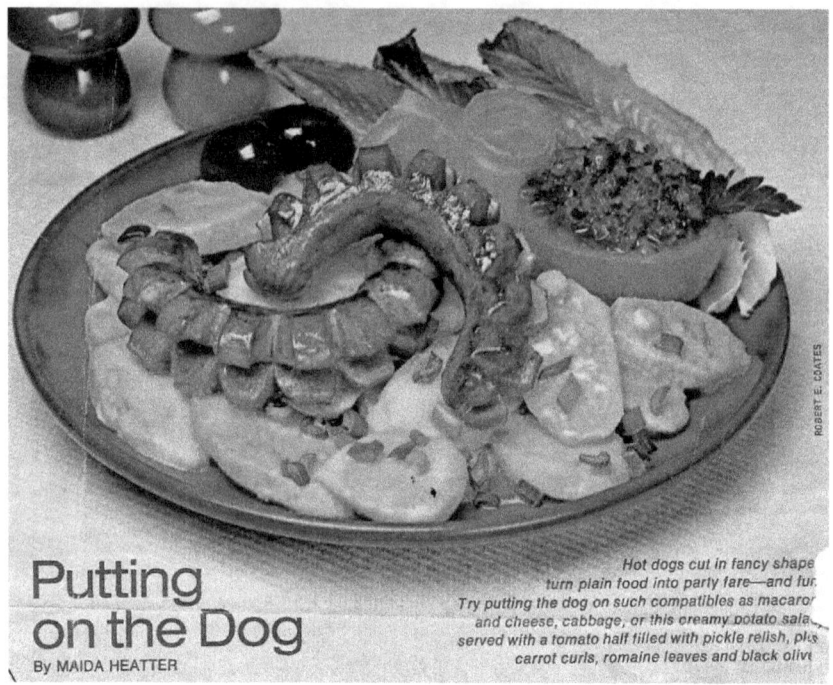

Coates

SPINAL TAP VERTEBRAE HOT DOGS

From the hair and the lyrics to the makeup – there's so much to love about the decadent lifestyle of 1980s heavy metal music. This Is Spinal Tap and here is a look at their hot dogs. Check out this interview of the band on what happened to Spinal Tap's First Drummer Stumpy Joe:

Marty DiBergi: *"What happened to Stumpy Joe?"*

Derek Smalls: *"It's not a very pleasant story. But uh, he died. He choked on uh, the official explanation was he choked on vomit."*

Nigel Tufnel: *"It was actually. It was actually someone else's vomit. You know there's no real..."*

Derek Smalls: *"Well they can't prove whose vomit it was. They don't have the ability. There's no way of..."*

Nigel Tufnel: *"You can't really dust for vomit."*

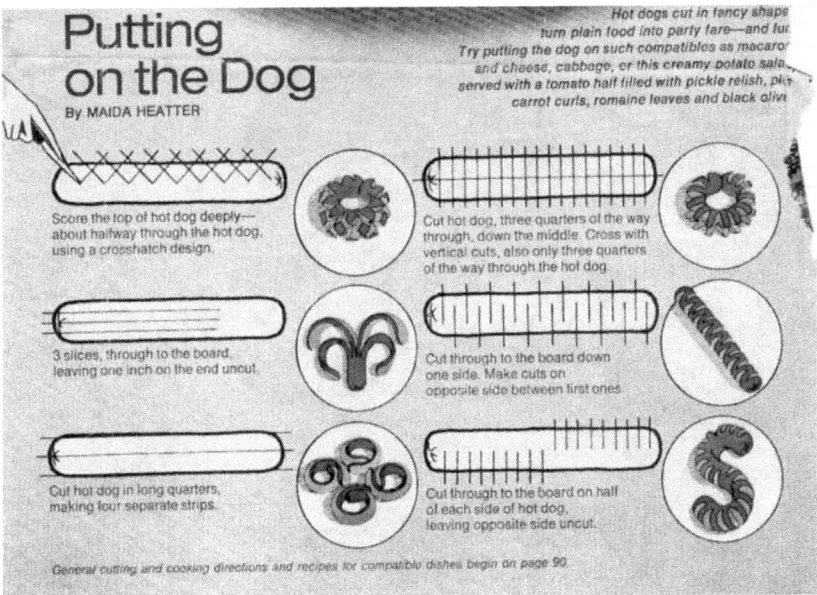

Coates

Instructions:
Cut your wiener up just like in the pictures above.

Cook 'em up and impress all your friends.

And you thought you'd figured out <u>all</u> the ways to have fun with your wiener!

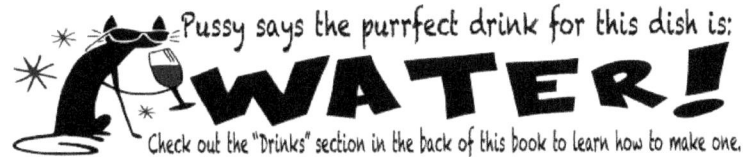

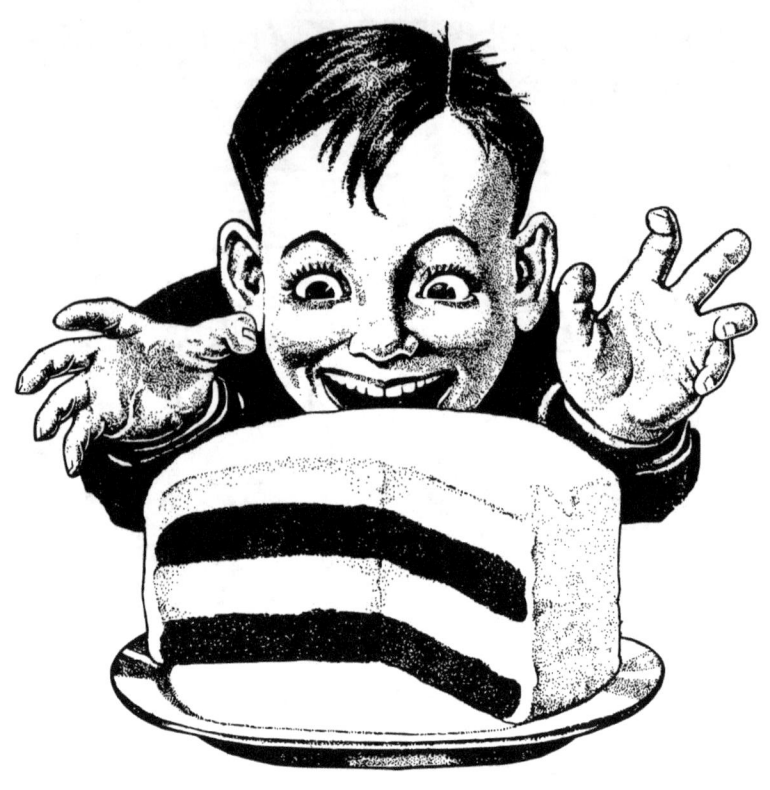

Deserts

After a long day of eating cock or whatever you've been shoving into your mouth, you may need some well-deserved relief.

Here are some recipes guaranteed to get any taste out of your mouth.

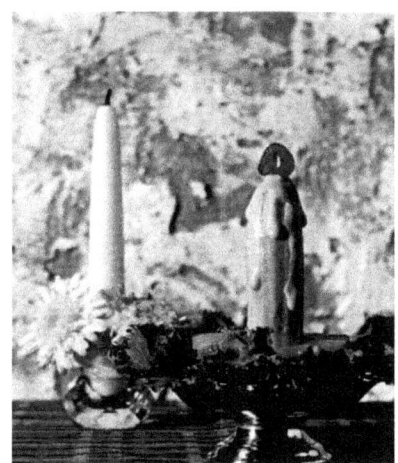

Banana Mayonnaise Candle

Ingredients:
3 bananas
2 tablespoons lemon juice
6 pineapple rings
2 tablespoons mayonnaise
3 glacé cherries

Instructions:
Halve the bananas crosswise, dip in lemon juice and place each half, end uppermost, in a pineapple ring. Drip mayonnaise down the sides of the bananas.

Using a toothpick, fix half a cherry on top of each banana. It will resemble a burning candle in its holder. Place each "candle" on a small plate, lined with lettuce leaves.

Orange slices can be used instead of pineapple rings. Serve up.

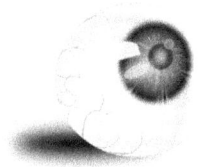

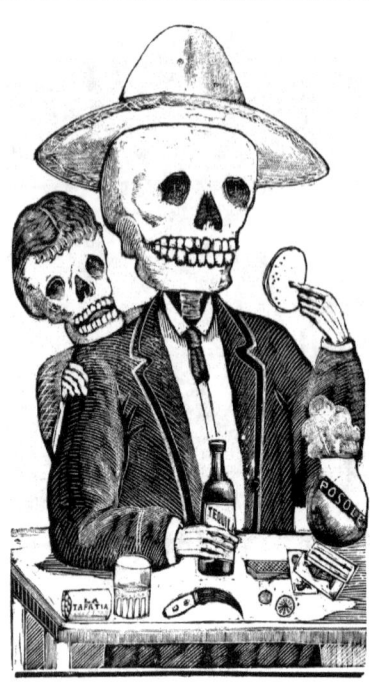

Tequila Cookies
Tequila Mockingbird
Ocean City, MD

Tequila. The classic that taste fantastic! Not only in our mouths but in just about anything, including cookies!

Ingredients:
1 bottle (edit) tequila (no worm!)
1 cup of dark brown sugar
1 cup (2 sticks) butter
1 cup of granulated sugar
4 large eggs
2 cups of dried fruit, such as dried cranberries or raisins
1 tsp baking soda
1 tsp salt
1 tsp fresh lemon juice
1 cup coarsely chopped walnuts or pecans
2 cups all-purpose flour

Instructions:
Sample the tequila often to check and recheck quality.

Take a large bowl, recheck the tequila to be sure it is of the highest quality. Pour one level cup and drink.

Turn on the electric mixer and beat one cup of butter in a large fluffy bowl.

Add one teaspoon of sugar...Beat again.

At this point, it's best to make sure the tequila is still okay, try another cup .... just in case.

Turn off the mixerer thingy. Break 2 leggs and add to the bowl and chuck in the cup of dried fruitz.

Pick the frigging fruit off floor... Mix on the turner. If the fried druit gets stuck in the beaterers just pry it loose with a drewscriver.

Sample the twiqulia to check for tonsisticity.

Next, sift two cops of salt, or something.

Check the Teeeqeeeya! I love you, man.

Now shift the lemon juz and strain yer nuts. Add one table. Get up off the floor and add a spoon of sugar, or somefink. Whatever you can find that has a pretty color and smellz good. I meen cookking iz art wight? I love yiu man!
Grease the oven. Turn the cake tin 360° and try not to fall over. Don't get tu turn beaterz off.

Finallllly, throo the bowl out the window. Who needs ookiez any ways?!

Finish the ... and make sure to put the stove in the dishwasher .... A dity stov iz not so good.

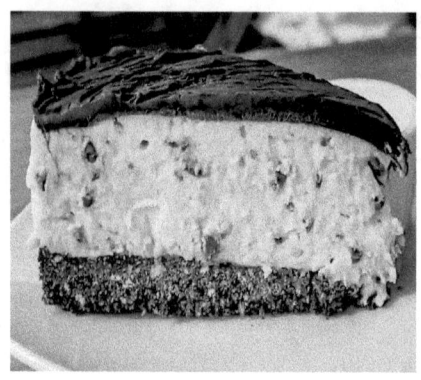

MILE HIGH ASPHALT PIE
DENVER MINT
DENVER, CO.

Munchies are just a way of life in Denver. They sell more food per capita than just about everyone. Hummm. I wonder why?

People agree that Mile High Asphalt Pie is so much better than any old flatlander cream pie! Too many blue ribbons to count. You need to say "sorry, thank you, let's get naked or all three, then show up with this pie!

Ingredients:

For Asphalt Pie:
24 Oreos crushed
4 Tbsp butter melted
1.5 quarts mint chocolate chip ice cream
(Double the ice cream for a MILE HIGH pie!)

For Salted Caramel:
1/2 cup sugar
3 Tbsp butter sliced
1/4 cup heavy cream
1/2 tsp sea salt
For Whipped Cream:
1 cup whipping cream
1/2 cup powdered sugar

Instructions:
 For Asphalt Pie:
Mix Oreos and melted butter. Stir until combined.

Eat some when no one is looking.

Press into the bottom of a pie pan.

Fill pie crust with ice cream. Cover and freeze for at least three hours before serving.

 For Salted Caramel:
Instructions:
 For Asphalt Pie:
Mix Oreos and melted butter. Stir until combined. Press into the bottom of a pie pan.

Fill pie crust with ice cream. Cover and freeze for at least three hours before serving.

 For Salted Caramel
Heat the sugar in a sauce pan over medium heat, stirring constantly and scraping the bottom. Sugar will melt into an amber liquid.

Once it is melted, add the butter.

Once the butter is melted, add the cream and boil for 1 minute.

Remove from heat and stir in sea salt.

 For Whipped Cream:
Mix cream and sugar until it forms stiff peaks.

Remove pie from freezer. Drizzle caramel topping over each slice and add whipped cream. Enjoy!

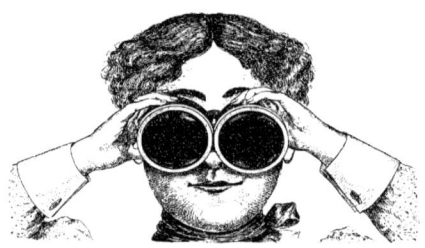

Now where is that damn waiter with our drinks?!

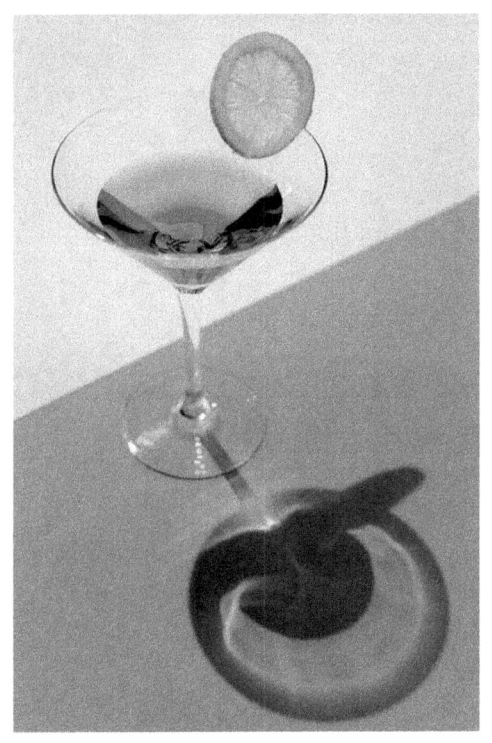

DRINKS

Buttery Nipple

Everybody loves a buttery nipple. The only thing better than a buttery nipple as a nipple with bacon. Here is the recipe for the nipple without the bacon.

Ingredients:
1 oz DeKuyper® Buttershots liqueur
1/2 oz Irish cream

Instructions:

Pour 1 oz of Buttershots liqueur into chilled shot glass
Gently pour the Irish cream liqueur over the back of the bar spoon to layer the two ingredients

Zip It Down Creamy Milky Surprise Energy Drink

This is a very popular creamy drink that you can make from Zipfizz energy powder. You can also mix alcohol into the mix to match the flavor of the powder. This will pick you up in give you a buzz both at the same time.

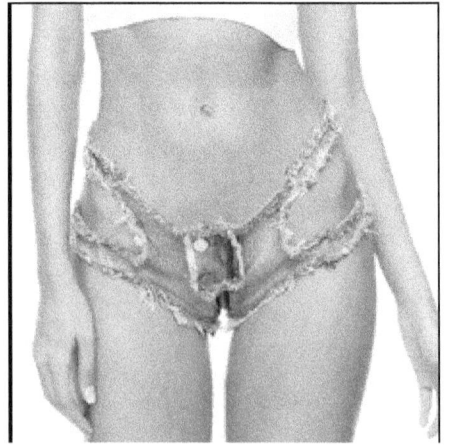

Ingredients:
1 Tube Zipfizz Energy Powder
1 1 oz coffee creamer
12 oz bottle of water

Instructions:
Open a cold 12 ounce bottle & drink about 2 ounces out of it.
Add small liquid coffee creamer.
Add tube of Zip Fizz Energy Powder.
Screw lid back on and shake.
Enjoy the creamy energy.

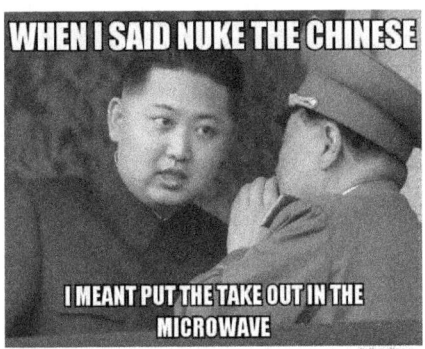

Purple-Headed Yogurt Flingers

Don't be afraid to experiment to see what combinations you like best, as it's difficult to make a bad Korean yogurt soju cocktail. It's delicious, refreshing, and tangy. But they can sneak up on you. So proceed with caution!

Ingredients:
3 ounces soju
3 ounces Asian yogurt drink (plain or flavored, thawed if frozen)
3 ounces lemon-lime soda (Sprite or 7 Up or fruit juice)

Instructions:

Into a stainless-steel cocktail shaker filled with ice, pour equal parts soju, yogurt drink, and soda.

Shake until ingredients are thoroughly chilled. Pour into a glass.

What Is Soju?
Soju is a common, highly potent alcohol in Korea. It's made by fermenting and then distilling a mixture that contains mainly rice and a blend of wheat, barley, and even sweet potatoes.

It is transparent and a mainly tasteless liquor, much like vodka and Kim Kardashian.

Sex on the Beach

The only thing worse than sex on the beach is sex in a cactus patch.

Ingredients:
1 1/2 oz vodka
1/2 oz peach schnapps
2 oz cranberry juice
2 oz orange juice

Instructions:
Add all the ingredients into a shaker with ice and shake. Strain into a highball glass over fresh ice.

Garnish with a cocktail umbrella.

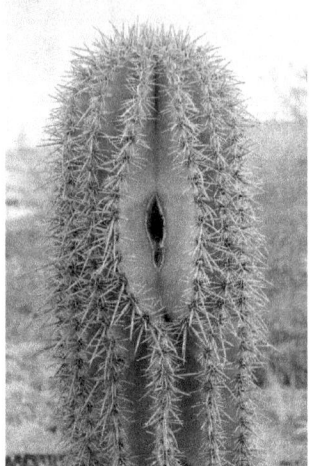

Blowjob

Blowjobs are great! Just do one at a time. No double dipping!

Ingredients:
1/4 oz Bailey's® Irish cream
1/2 oz amaretto almond liqueur

Instructions:
Add all the ingredients into a shaker with ice and shake hard. Be careful not to spill a drop.

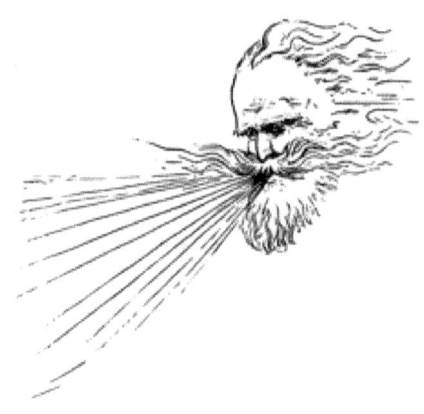

Liquid Viagra

When you cant get it going at the local bar this drink will get you up!

Ingredients:
1 shot Jägermeister herbal liqueur
1/3 can Red Bull energy drink

Instructions:
Pour red bull into a large glass. Drop a shot of Jägermeister, including the shot glass, into the red bull and lift it up to your mouth.

Slippery Nipple

What is more fun for everyone then slippery nipples?

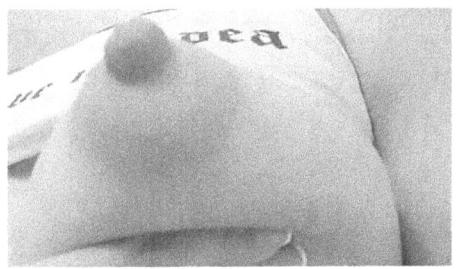

Ingredients:
1/2 oz Bailey's® Irish cream
1/2 oz butterscotch schnapps

Instructions:
No instructions needed. You have known what to do with those since you were born!

Screaming Orgasm

The perfect thing to wake up her mom and dad sleeping in the bedroom next door while visiting them on vacation!

Ingredients:
1 oz vodka
1 1/2 oz Bailey's Irish cream
1/2 oz Kahlua coffee liqueur

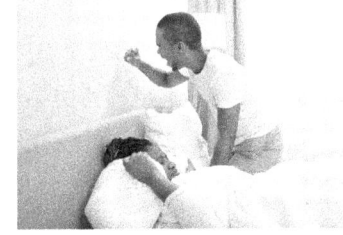

Instructions:
If you slam it all hard enough, she may forget where she is at!

Super Slow Comfortable Screw

Incredibly easy to make and hard to screw up. If you can mix up a screwdriver, this drink's the same thing. It is definitely the most popular sloe gin cocktail and a fun retro drink.

Ingredients:
1 oz sloe gin
1/2 oz Southern Comfort® peach liqueur
orange juice

Instructions:
Fill a highball glass with ice and pour in the sloe gin and the peach licker. Top it up with orange juice and garnish with an orange slice if you feel fancy!

Sex Machine

A great drink to enjoy when you are home alone with the power on!

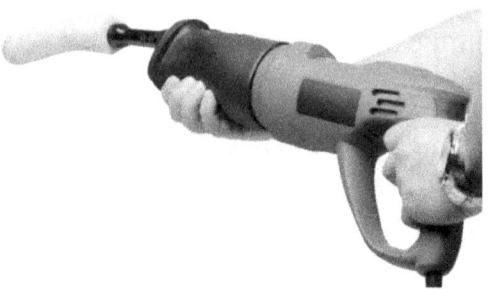

Ingredients:
1.5 oz. Bailey's,
1.5 oz. Kahlua,
1.5 oz. Milk.

Instructions:
Put 1-2 ice cubes in a glass, pour the liqueurs. Hold back the milk until you can't stand it anymore, and then let it go.

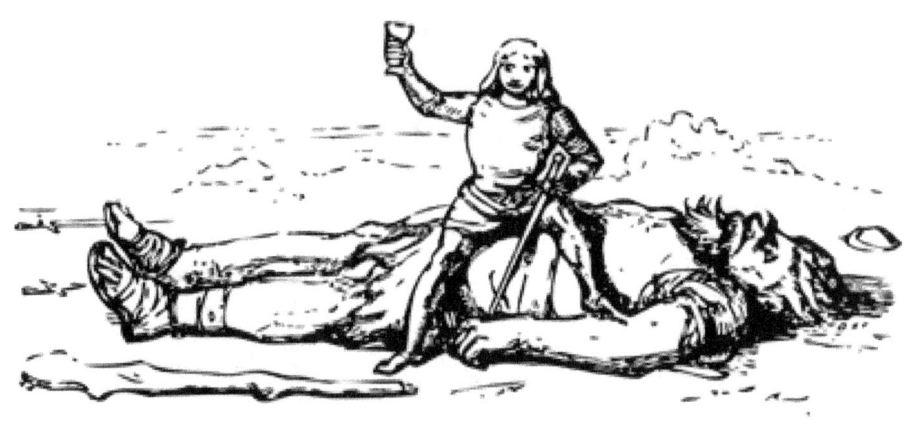

Sit on My Face

Ingredients:
1/3 oz Kahlua coffee liqueur
1/3 oz Frangelico hazelnut liqueur
1/3 oz Bailey's Irish cream

Instructions:

Pour the Coffee Liqueur into a Shot Glass
Add in the Hazelnut Liqueur
Float the Irish Cream on top

Deep Throat

Ingredients:
1/2 oz Bailey's Irish cream
1/2 oz Kahlua coffee liqueur
1/2 oz whipped cream

Instructions:
In a cocktail glass add the Irish cream, coffee liqueur and you know what to do with the cream.

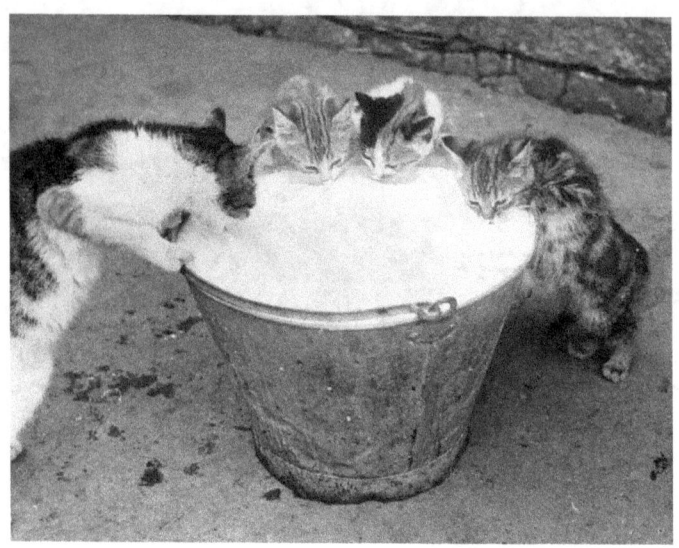

Creamy Pussy

Ingredients:
1 oz Bailey's® Irish cream
1 oz Tequila Rose® strawberry cream liqueur

Instructions:

Combine ingredients together and share your cream with friends.

Harvey Wall banger
Ingredients:
1.5 oz Smirnoff No. 21 Vodka
0.25 oz hazelnut liqueur
3 oz orange juice
1 slice orange

Instructions:

Combine all ingredients into a thermos and shake. Go to an adult book store and stick your finger through the hole in the wall. Wait for Harvey to stick through it. Don't forget to bang on the wall before coming!

Pop My Cherry

Ingredients:
1/2 oz cherry vodka
1/4 oz triple sec
1/4 oz orange juice

Instructions:
Combine ingredients into a cocktail glass and stir rapidly.

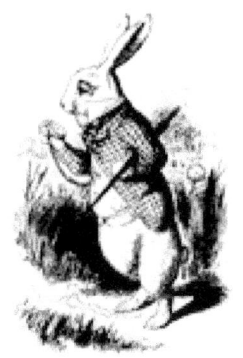

Bend Over Shirley

Ingredients:
1 1/2 oz raspberry vodka
4 oz Sprite® soda
3/4 oz Rose's® grenadine syrup

Instructions:
Fill a 12oz. glass with cubed ice. Add 1.5 oz. of Raspberry Vodka. Add Sprite, and top off with Grenadine. Garnish with two Maraschino Cherries.

Three-Legged Monkey

Ingredients:
1 oz Crown Royal® Canadian whisky
1 oz amaretto almond liqueur
1 oz pineapple juice

Instructions:
Pour Crown, Amaretto and pineapple juice in to a Shaker with ice. Shake until really cold. Pour into shot glass and serve.

DR. PECKER

Ingredients:
2 oz Rye Whiskey
2 oz Cola
2 oz Cranberry-Raspberry Juice

Instructions:
Stir ingredients together in a highball glass filled with ice cubes, and serve.

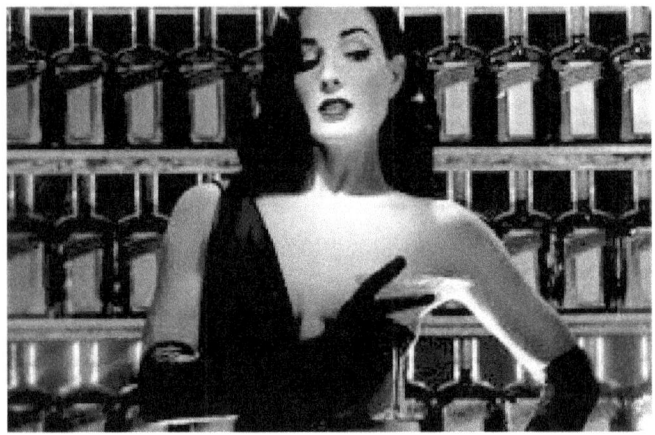

PENILE COLAROUS

Ingredients:
1/4 oz Banana Liqueur
1/2 oz Coconut Rum
1/4 oz Peach Schnapps
1/4 oz Pina Colada Schnapps
3 oz Pineapple Juice

Instructions:
When shaken properly it provokes the desire, but it takes away the performance.

Tight Snatch

Everyone enjoys a good properly prepared Tight Snatch!

Ingredients:
Ice
1 shot vodka
1 shot peach schnapps
orange juice
cranberry juice

Instructions:
Shake with ice. Serve in ice-filled glass.

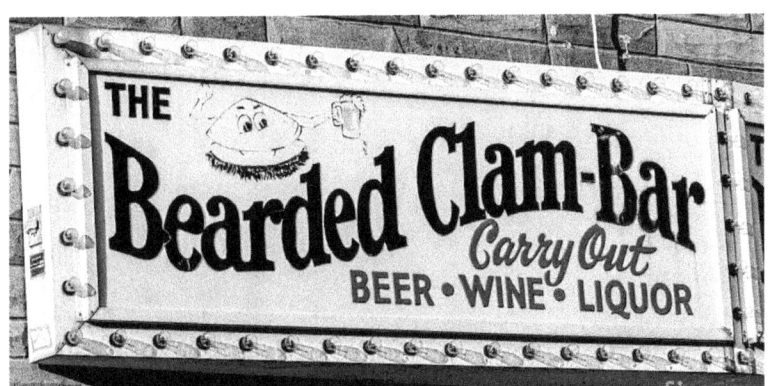

Bearded Clam
Ingredients:
1 oz. Crown Royal
1 oz. Amaretto
1 splash Cranberry Juice

Instructions:
Shake with ice. Serve in ice-filled glass.

Strawberry Stripper
Ingredients:
5 oz. Orange Juice
1 oz. 7-Up
1 splash(es) Grenadine
1 oz. Strawberry Schnapps

Instructions:
Shake with ice. Serve in ice-filled glass.

Orange Bush
Question: What happened when Donald Trump got drunk with Barbra Bush in the 1980's?

Answer: Trump quit drinking!

Ingredients:
1/4 oz. Vodka
1 oz. Orange Juice

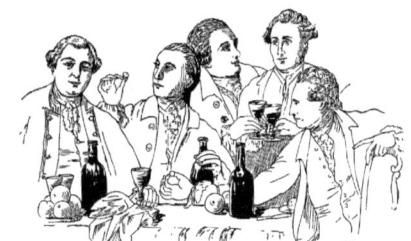

Instructions:
Shake with ice. Serve in ice-filled glass.

Fuzzy Navel
Ingredients:
1 part peach schnapps
1 part orange juice
1 part lemonade

Instructions:
Shake with ice. Serve in ice-filled glass.

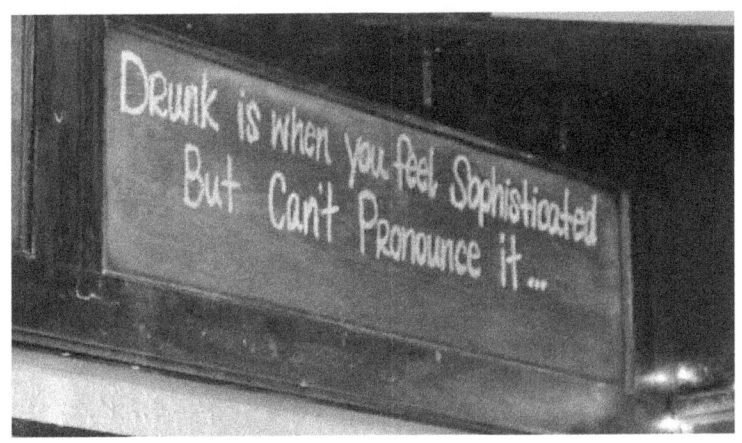

Dirty Mother

Ingredients:
1 1/2 oz brandy
1/2 oz Kahlua® coffee liqueur

Instructions:
Shake with ice. Serve in ice-filled glass.

Golden Shower

Ingredients:
1 oz Stolichnaya® vodka
1 oz orange juice
1/2 oz fresh lemon juice
1 splash triple sec
ginger ale

Instructions:
Shake with ice. Serve in ice-filled glass.
.

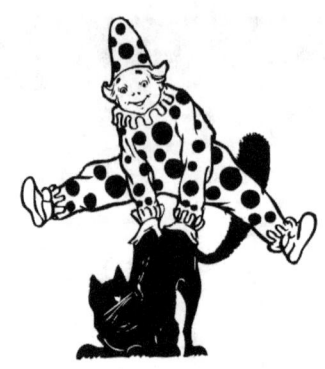

Super Red Balls

Ingredients:
1 1/2 oz pomegranate vodka
1 oz coconut rum
1 oz crème de almond
1/2 oz sweet vermouth
dash of lime juice
maraschino cherry for garnish

Instructions:
Shake with ice. Serve in ice-filled glass.

Royal Fook

Ingredients:
2 parts Crown Royal
1 part Sour Apple Pucker
1 part Cranberry Juice

Instructions:
Shake with ice. Serve in ice-filled glass.

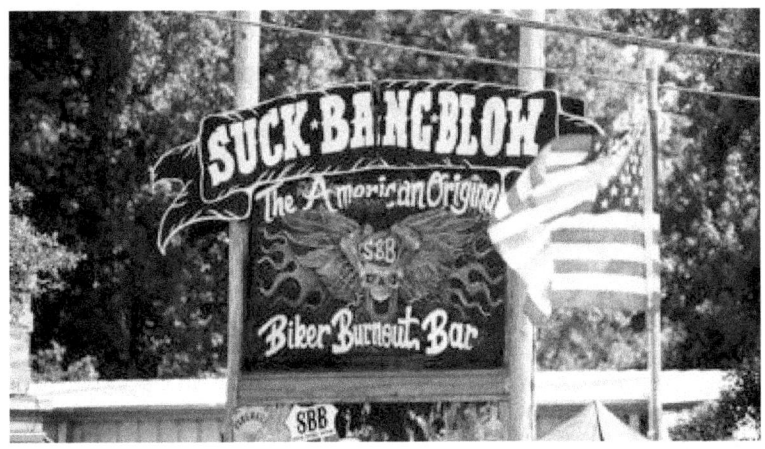

Suck, Bang and Blow

Something bikers should probably share only with their female friends if they want to make it out the door alive at the Biker Burnout Bar in Murrells Inlet South Carolina!

Ingredients:
1 oz Jacquin's orange Flavored gin
1 oz Rumple Minze
2 oz Gold schlager
1 oz Jägermeister
3 oz Jose Cuervo Especial gold tequila
1 oz Smirnoff vodka
1 oz Absolut citron
1 oz Aristocrat triple sec
1 peeled, whole lime
5 oz Strawberry Daiquiri Mix
2 cups cranberry juice
1 cup sugar

Instructions:
Add all ingredients to a blender with ice, and blend until smooth. Pour into a hurricane glass, and serve.

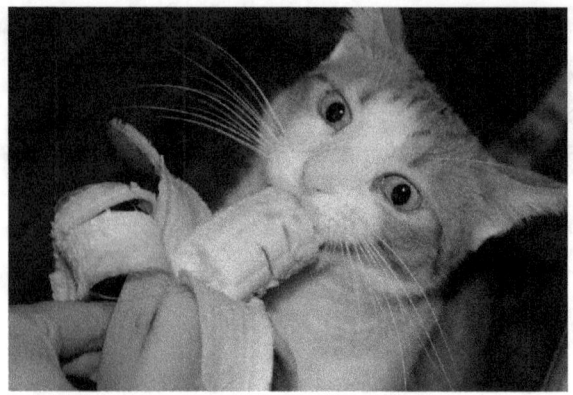

kittentoob

How to Eat Pussy

Everyone loves some good cock. Am I right? I mean cock that has been simmering all day. You can smell the cock for blocks around. I know I smell hot cock and my mouth begins to water, and I imagine stuffing that cock into my mouth and swallowing it all. Now that you've got through this book, you can do the same any time you want! And if you do get tired of eating cock, you can always buy …

How to Eat Pussy
The Sofa King Easy Way!

Coming soon!

Bye-bye!

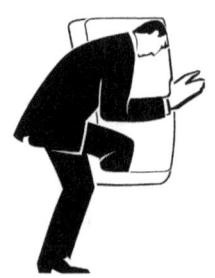

Copyrigt © 2020, Sofa King Rad, LLC
All Rights Reserved.

www.ingramcontent.com/pod-product-compliance
Lightning Source LLC
LaVergne TN
LVHW051550070426
835507LV00021B/2500